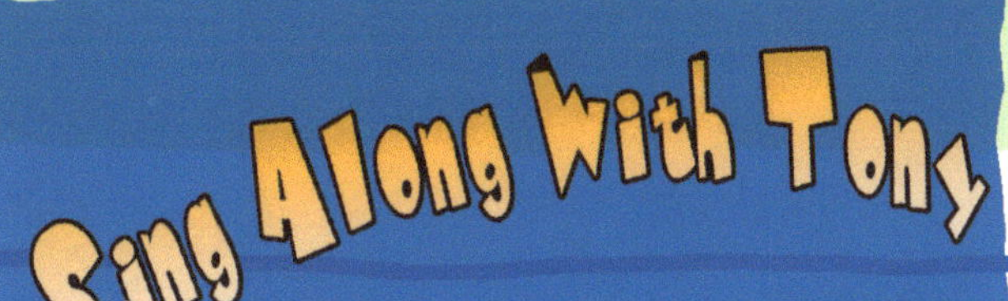

CROSSING THE MIDLINE

DANCES, ACTIVITIES AND EXERCISES

A resource for teachers, instructors and families

CONTENTS

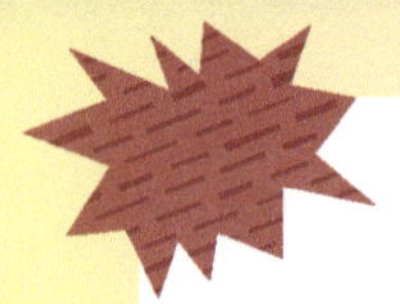

CONTENTS

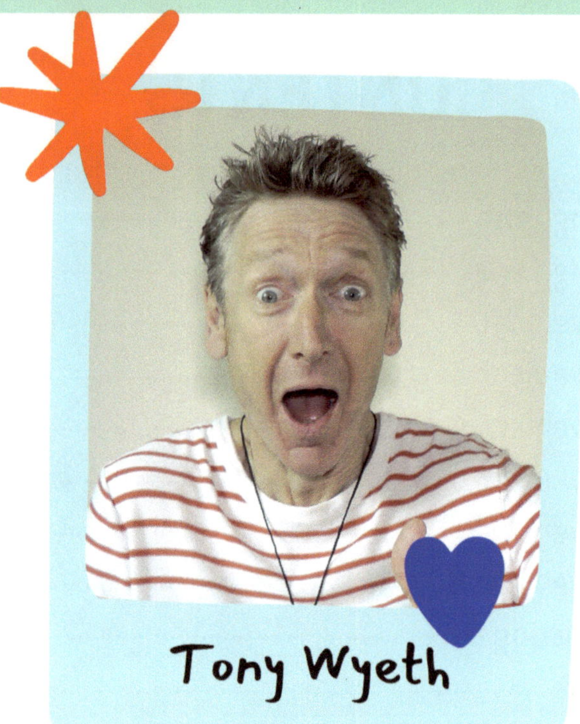

INTRODUCTION

Hello my beautiful friends!
My name is Tony and I like to sing and dance.
This book is a collection of dances, activities and exercises all designed to help you cross the midline.

The dances were created for my interactive live show **"Crossing the Midline"**.
The songs are from the Sing Along With Tony album **"Little Carrot's Friends"**,
available on SPOTIFY and all your favourite platforms.

If you would like more free resources or to get in touch, you can sign-up for news on my website here:
https://singalongwithtony.com/join-the-community/
Have fun!

WHAT IS CROSSING THE MIDLINE?

"Crossing the Midline" is a motor skill. It refers to the ability to reach across an imaginary line down the middle of the body, with the arms, hands, feet or legs, to perform a task.

It means the right and left sides of the brain must work together, hopefully in a coordinated manner. This is an important skill for the development of a variety of cognitive and motor skills.

In the classroom, reading and writing require crossing the midline. At home, simple tasks such as putting on shoes and socks require crossing the midline.

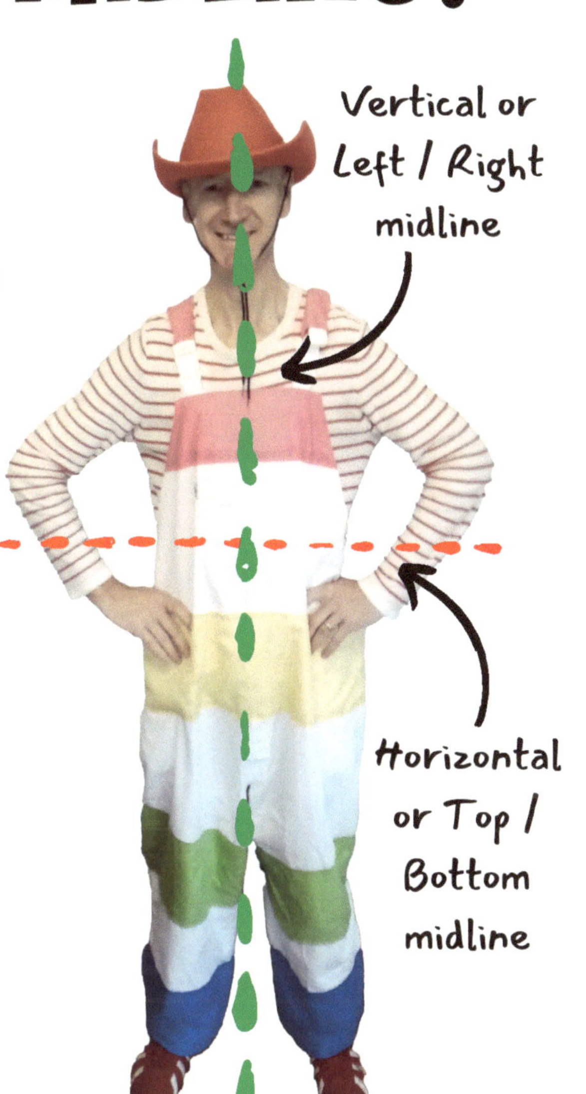

EXAMPLES OF CROSSING THE MIDLINE

Like this...

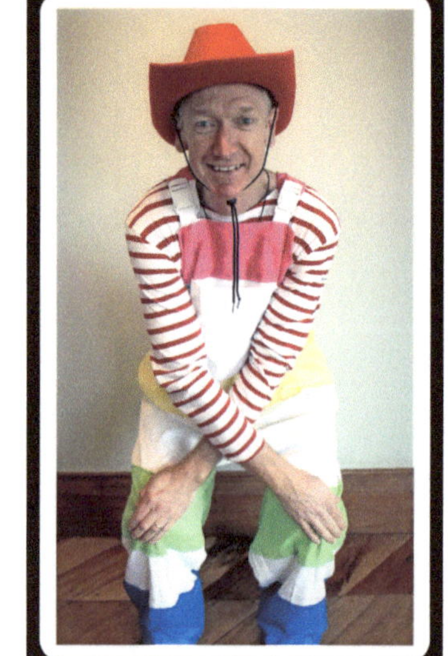

And this...

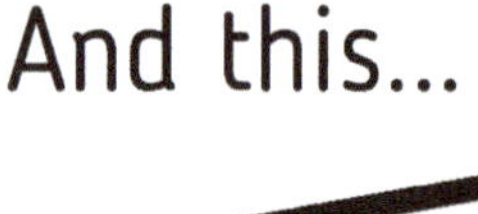

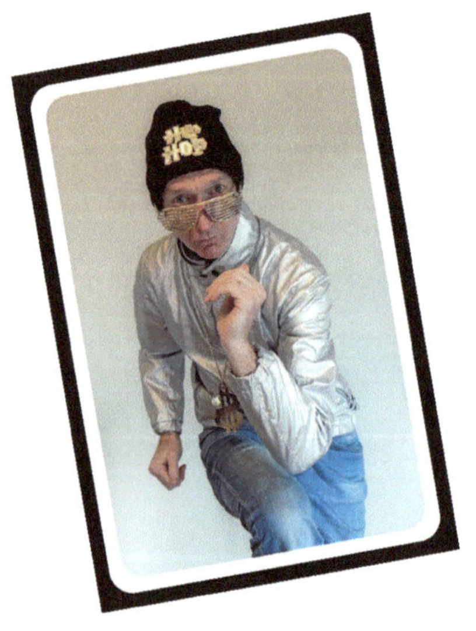

And this...

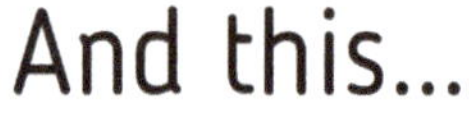

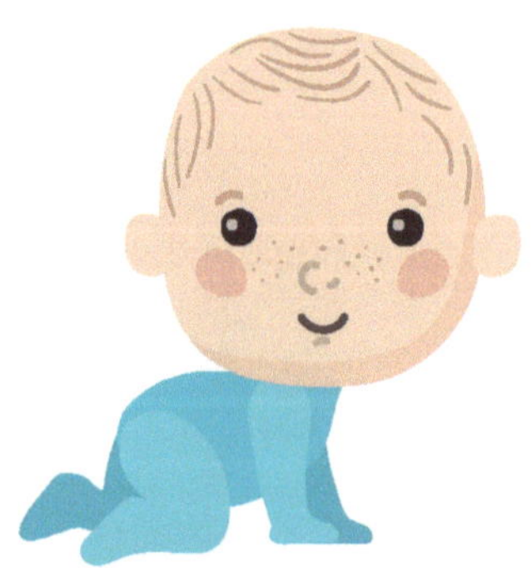

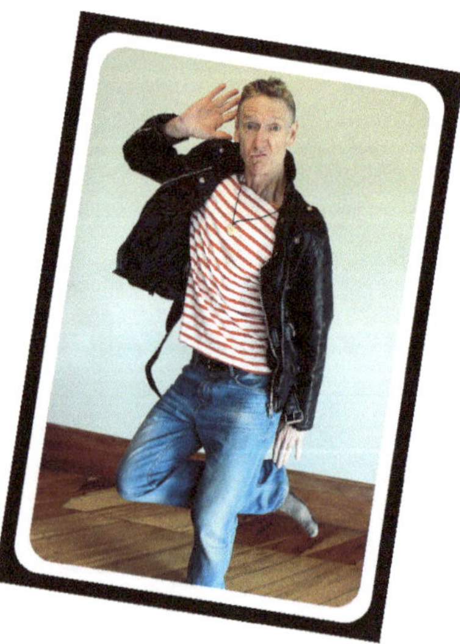

WHY IS CROSSING THE MIDLINE IMPORTANT?

Crossing the midline helps us :

- Develop a dominant hand
- Develop gross and fine motor skills
- Increase motor coordination
- Move from both sides of our body
- Know the right and left sides of our body

Children who have trouble crossing the midline often lose their place while reading or writing, making many school activities very difficult.

They may also struggle to draw shapes, such as "+" or "x" as easily or quickly as their classmates do.

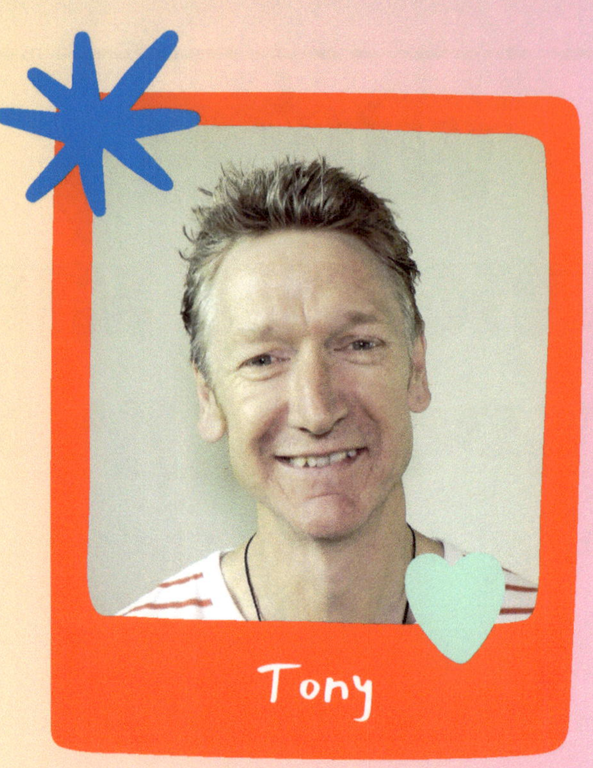

DANCE 1

The first dance we're going to learn is with my friend
Little Tomato.

Little Tomato sings a song about colours.
What is your favourite colour?

There's a photo of Little Tomato on the next page...

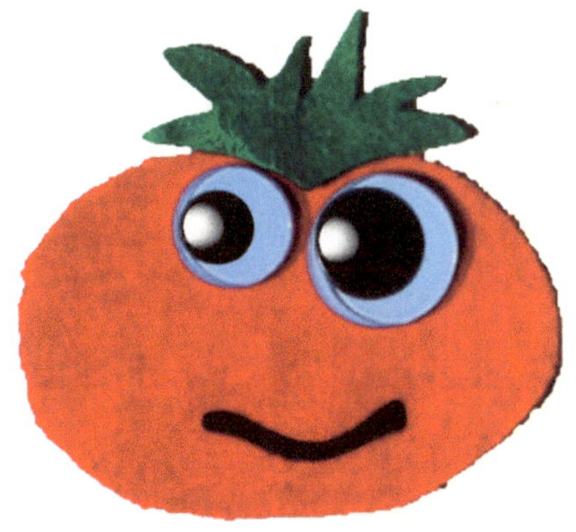

Little Tomato loves colours!
Will you sing and dance with him?

Little Tomato:
Colours

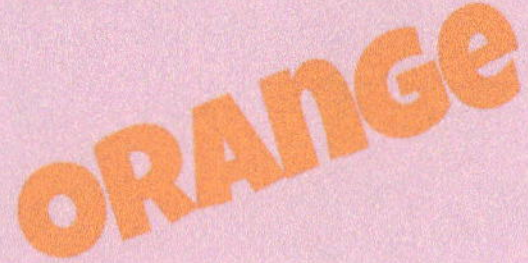

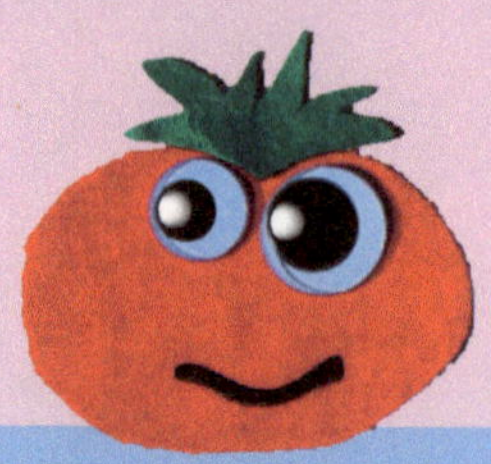

Little Tomato: Colours

What's your favourite colour, Little Tomato?
What's your favourite colour, Little Tomato?
My favourite colour is blue... blue, blue, blue, blue.
Blue, blue, blue, blue, my favourite colour is blue!

What's your favourite colour, Little Tomato?
What's your favourite colour, Little Tomato?
My favourite colour is green... green, green, green, green.
Green, green, green, green, my favourite colour is green!

What's your favourite colour, Little Tomato?
What's your favourite colour, Little Tomato?
My favourite colour is yellow... yellow, yellow.
Yellow, yellow, my favourite colour is yellow!

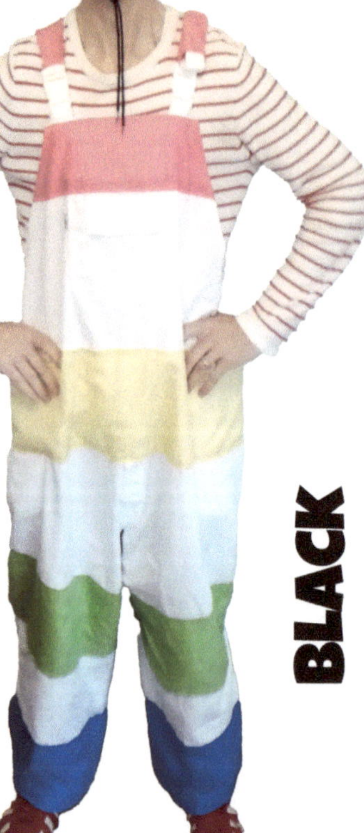

What's your favourite colour, Little Tomato?
What's your favourite colour, Little Tomato?
My favourite colour is pink... pink, pink pink, pink.
Pink, pink, pink, pink, my favourite colour is pink!

What's your favourite colour, Little Tomato?
What's your favourite colour, Little Tomato?
My favourite colour is red... red, red, red, red.
Red, red, red, red, my favourite colour is red!
Of course! I'm a tomato!

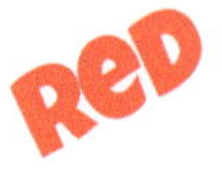

7

LITTLE TOMATO DANCE

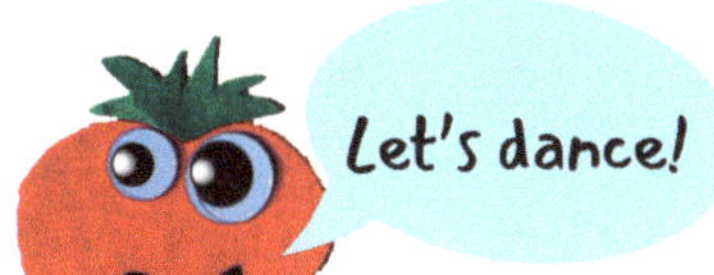

This dance involves 2 movements.

Movement 1
WALKING ON THE SPOT

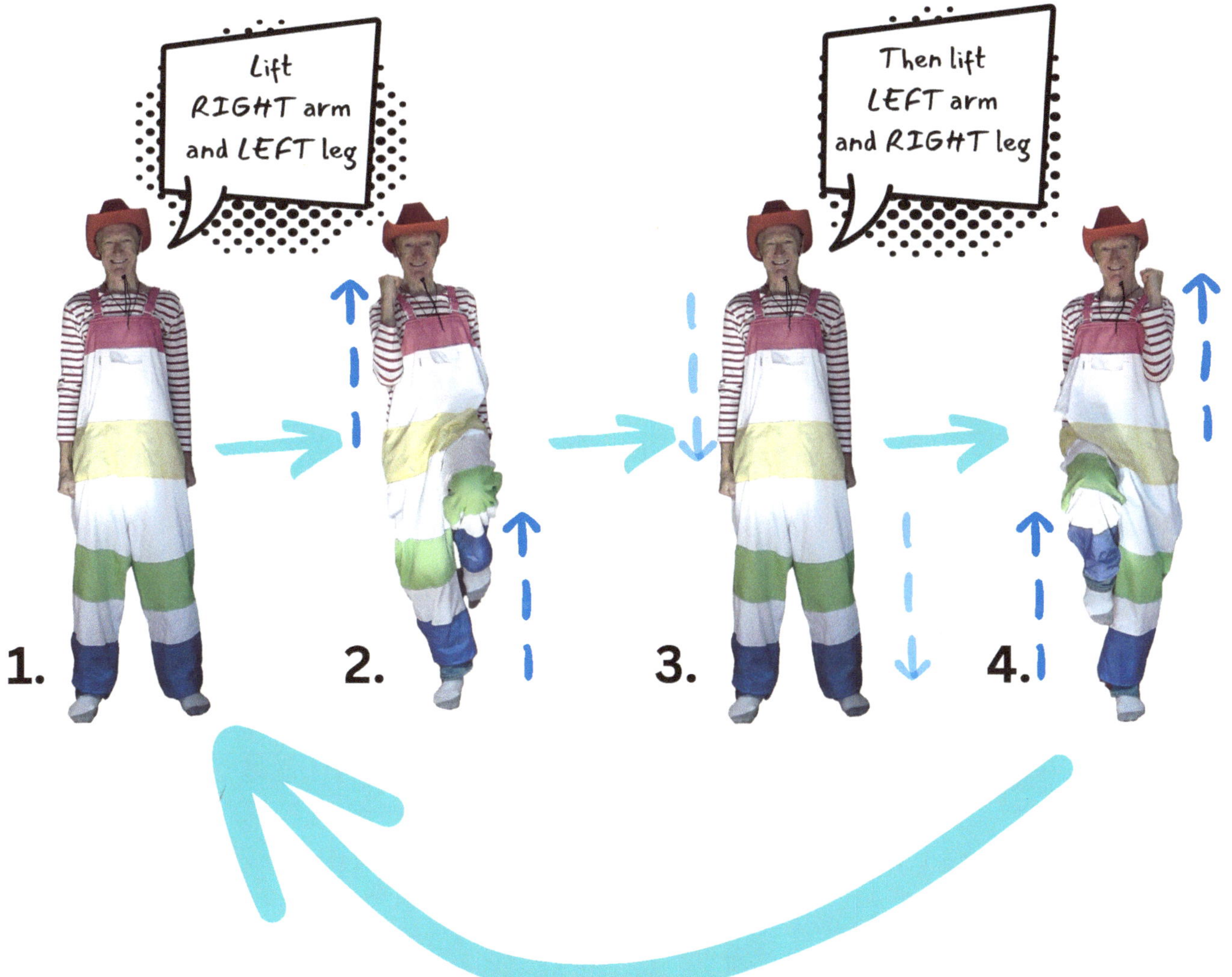

1.   2.   3.   4.

LITTLE TOMATO DANCE

Movement 1
WALKING ON THE SPOT

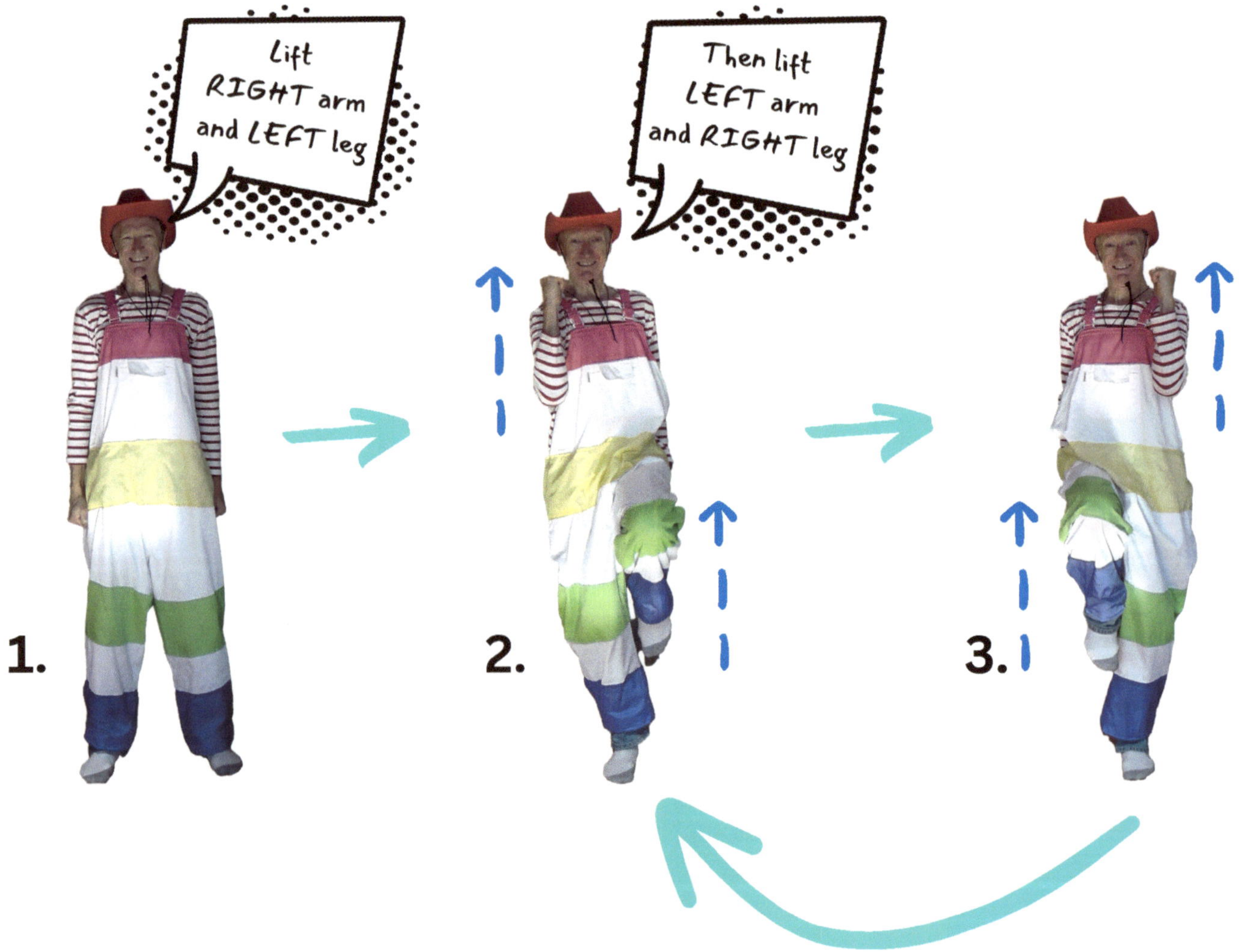

1.

2.

3.

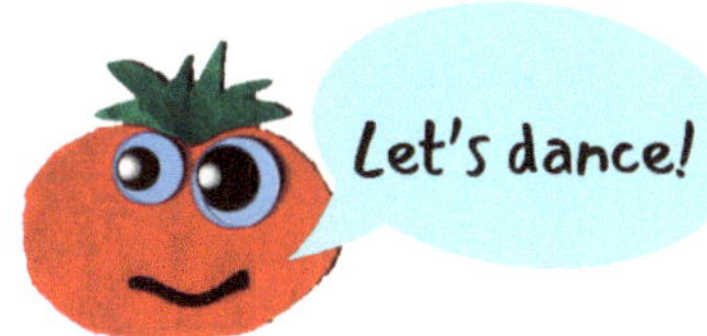

Movement 2
POINTING TO COLOURS

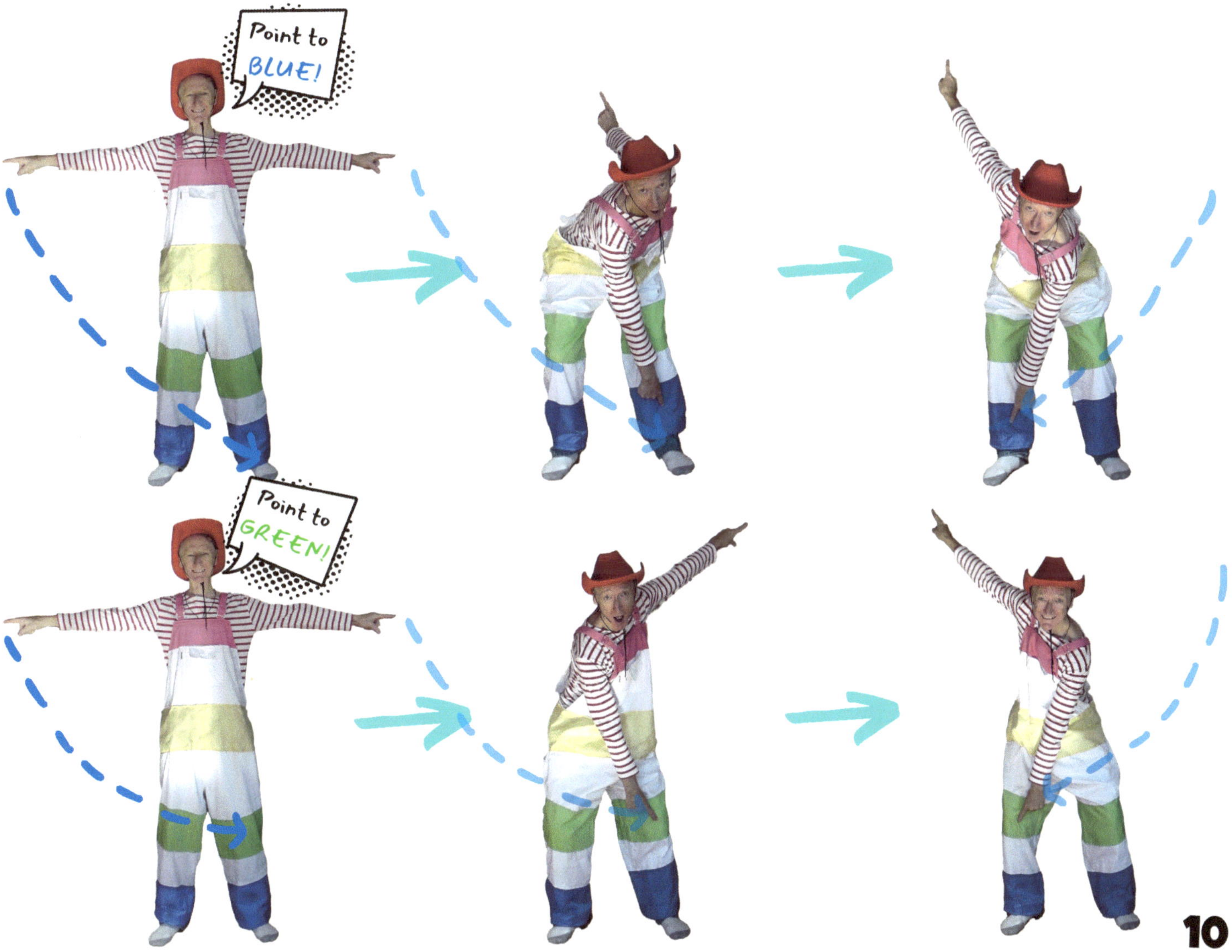

LITTLE TOMATO DANCE

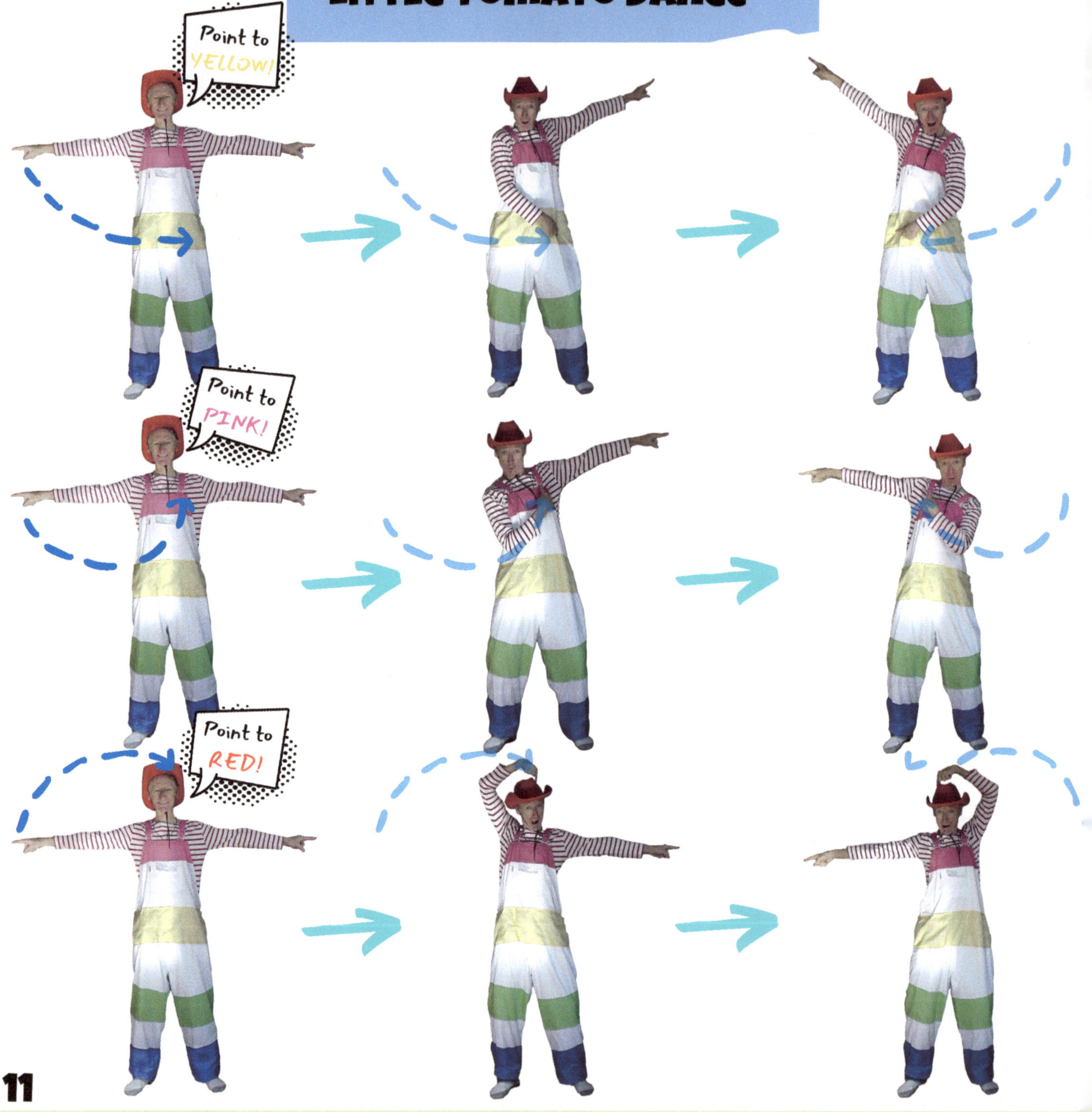

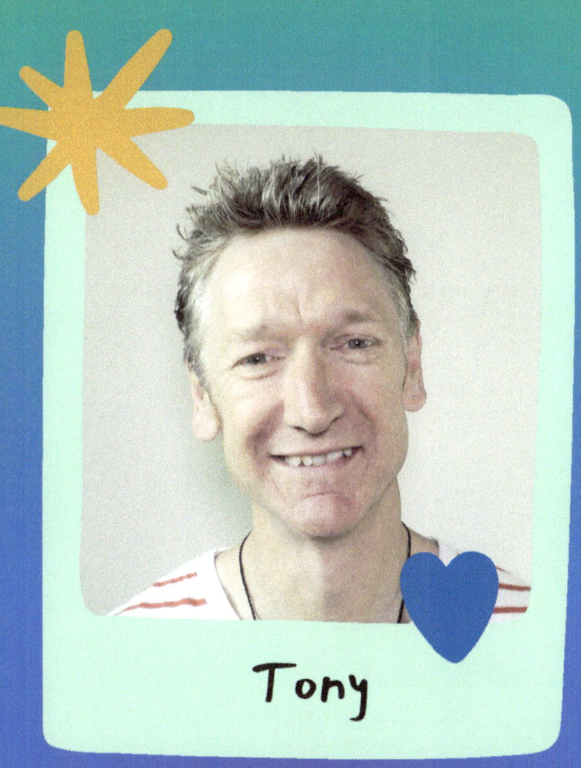

DANCE 2

Yay! That was cool!

The next dance we're going to learn is with my friend **Little Apple.**

Little Apple sings a song about the body.
Little Apple has hair, eyes, a nose...

There's a photo of Little Apple on the next page...

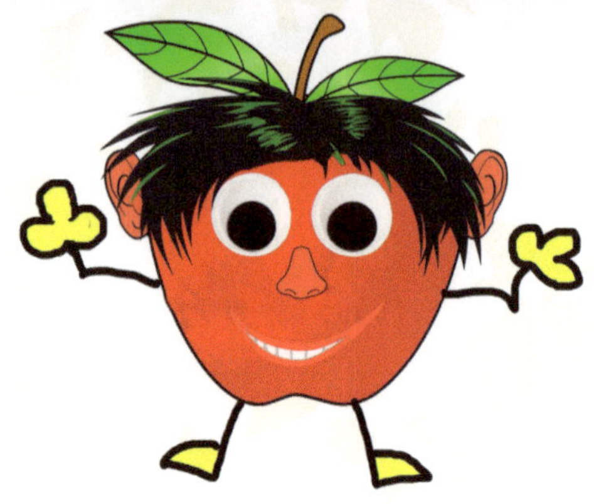

Little Apple has a mouth!
Let's sing and dance with him!

Little Apple:
The Body

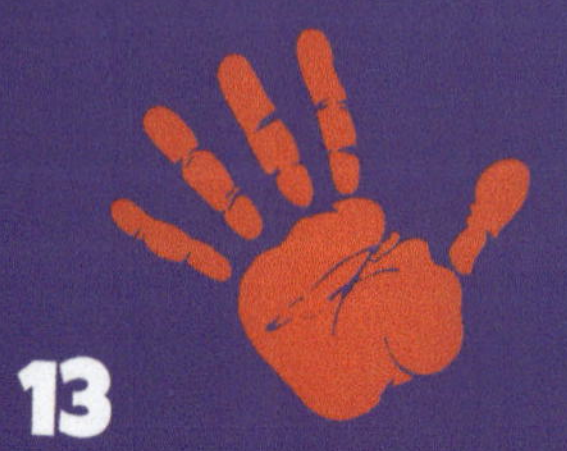

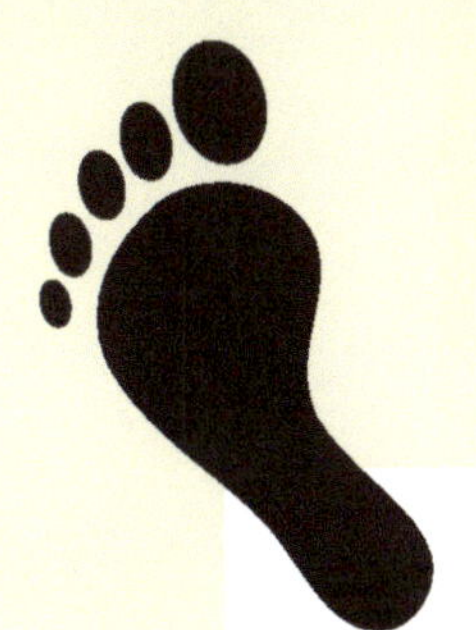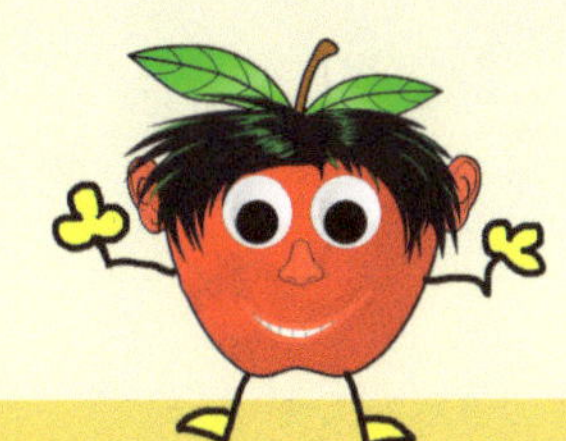

<u>Little Apple: The Body</u>

Look at me, I'm an apple! } *CHORUS*
Look at me, I'm an apple!

Where is your mouth, where is your mouth?
Look, look, look, it's my mouth.
Where is your eye, where is your eye?
Look, look, look, it's my eye.

CHORUS

Where is your nose, where is your nose?
Look, look, look, it's my nose.
Where is your ear, where is your ear?
Look, look, look, it's my ear.

CHORUS + INSTRUMENTAL

Where is your hair, where is your hair?
Look, look, look, it's my hair.
Where is your hand, where is your hand?
Look, look, look, it's my hand.

CHORUS (repeat)

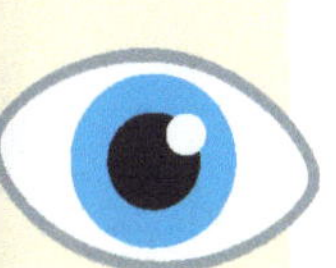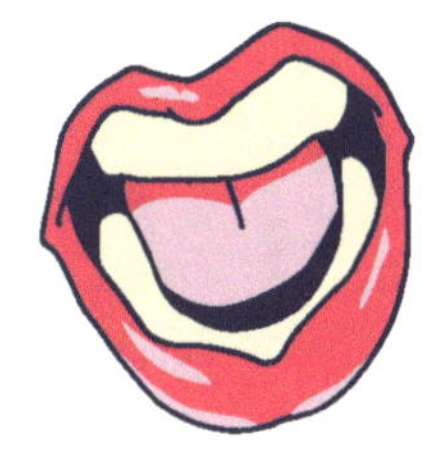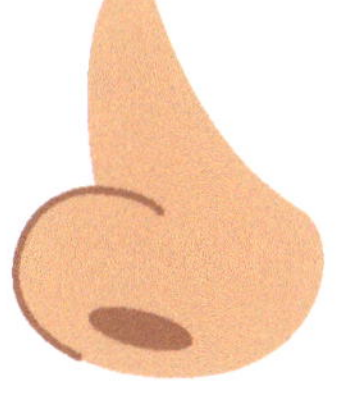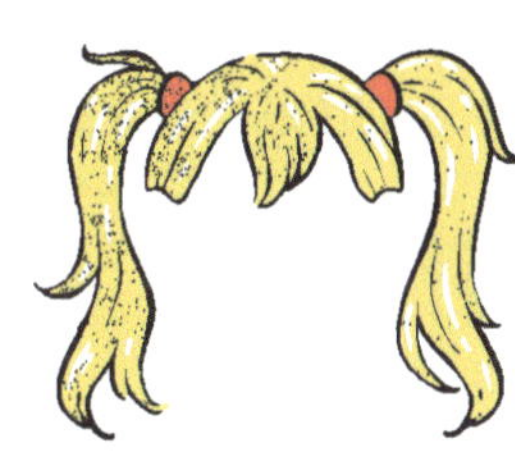

LITTLE APPLE DANCE

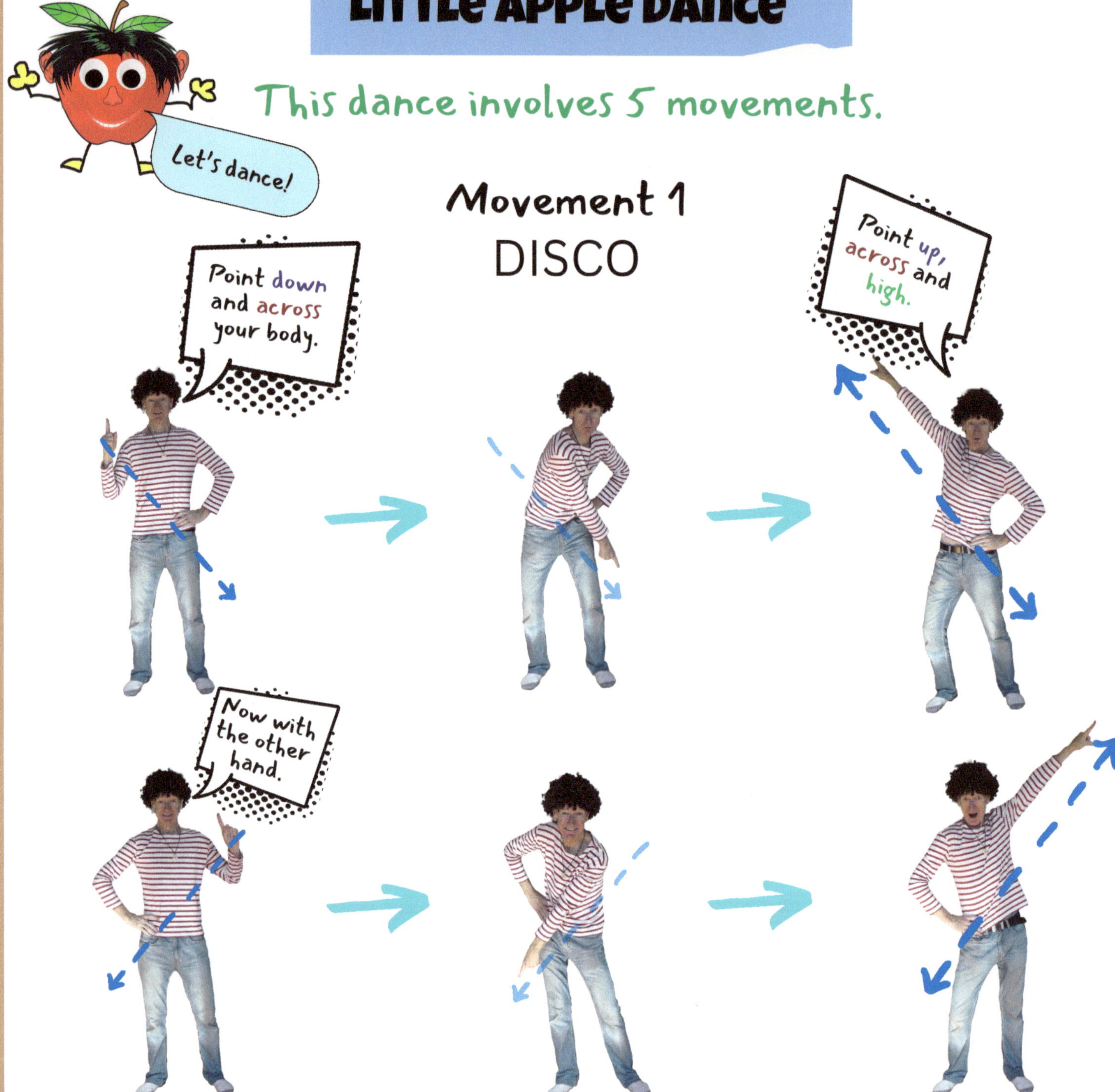

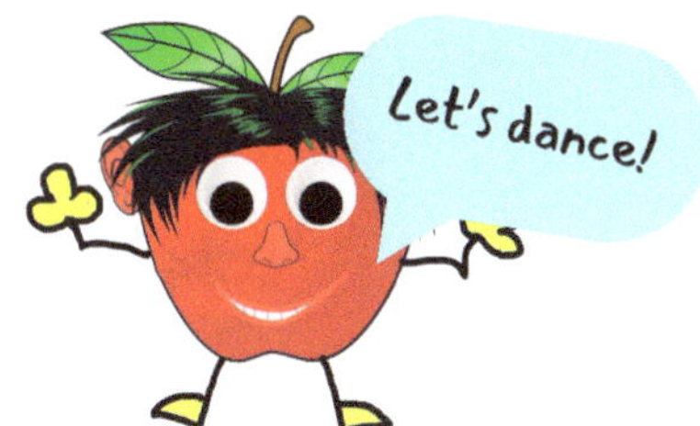

Movement 2
LOOK AT ME

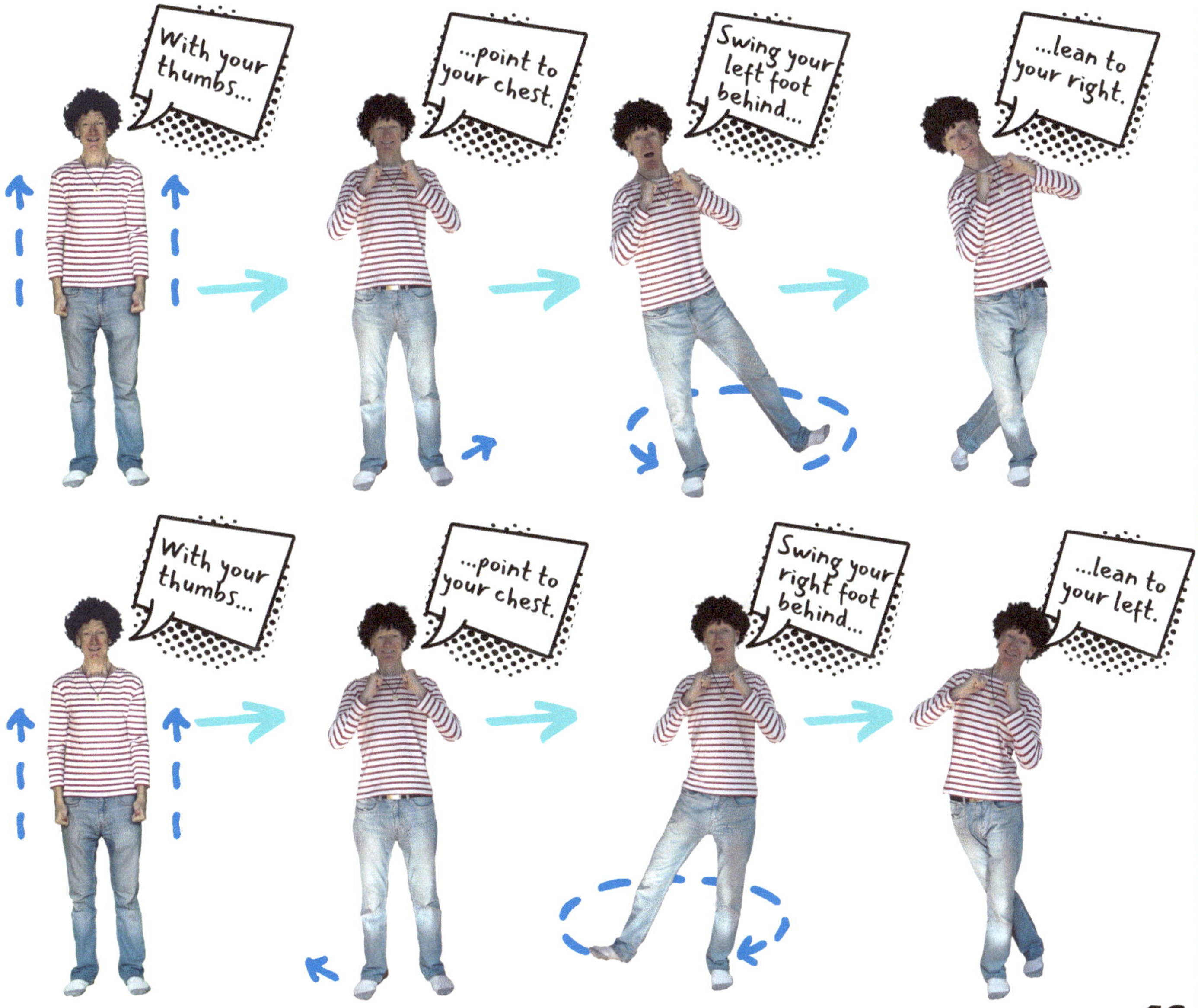

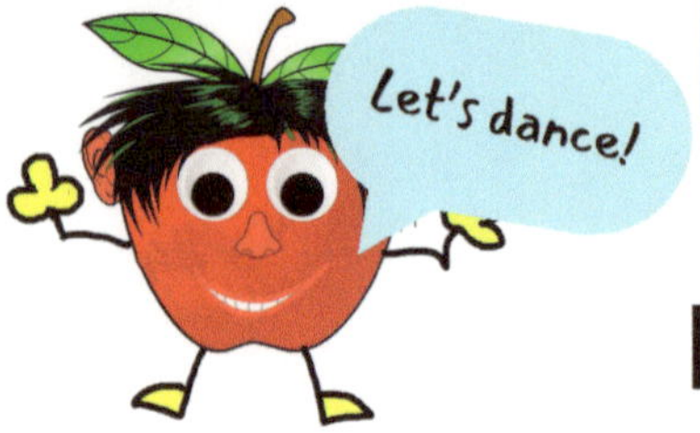

Movement 3
POINT TO BODY PARTS

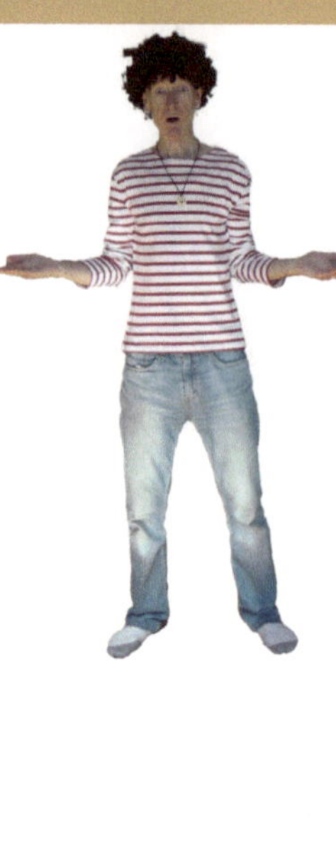

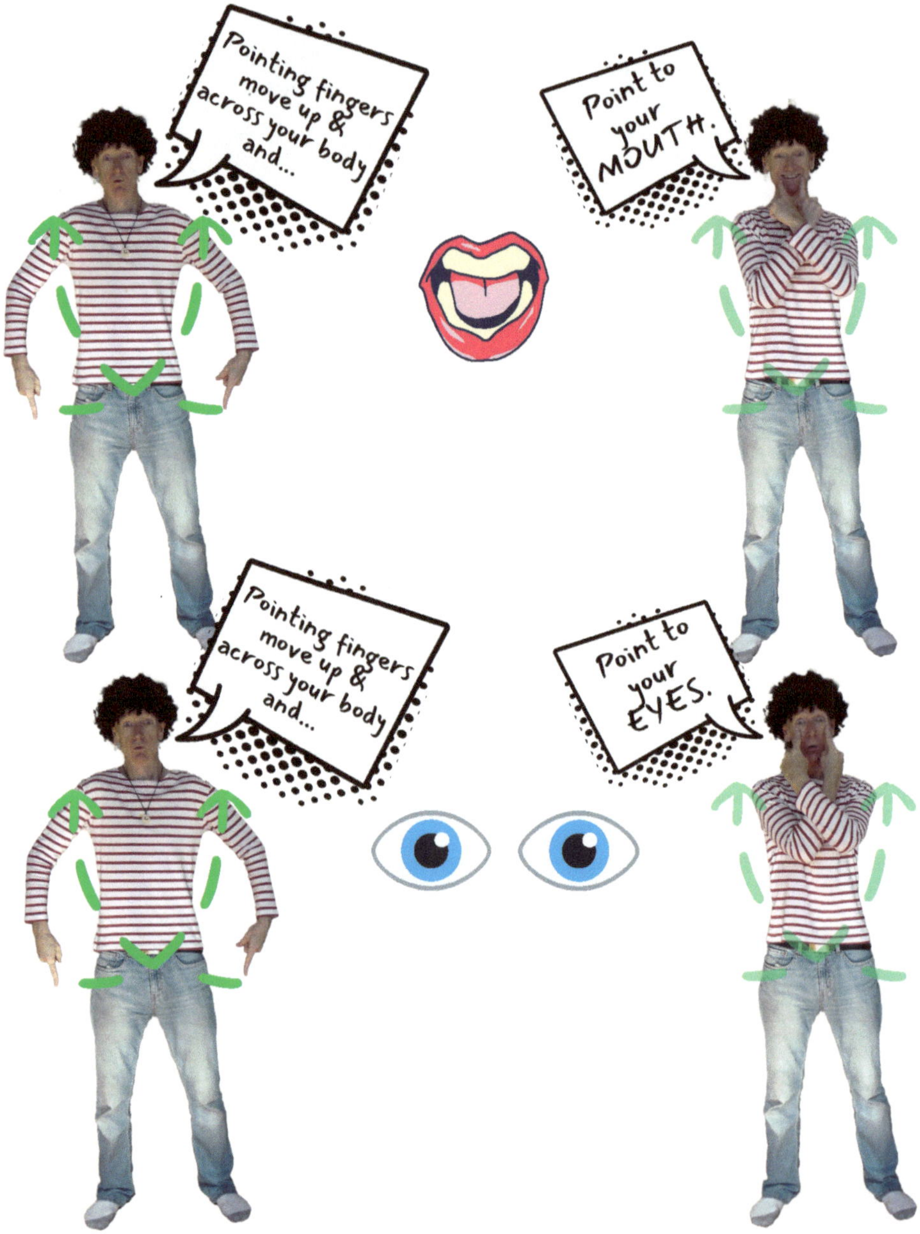

17

LITTLE APPLE DANCE

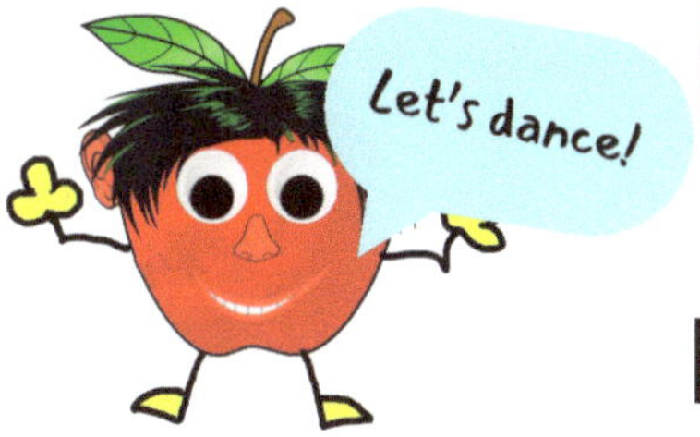

Movement 3
POINT TO BODY PARTS

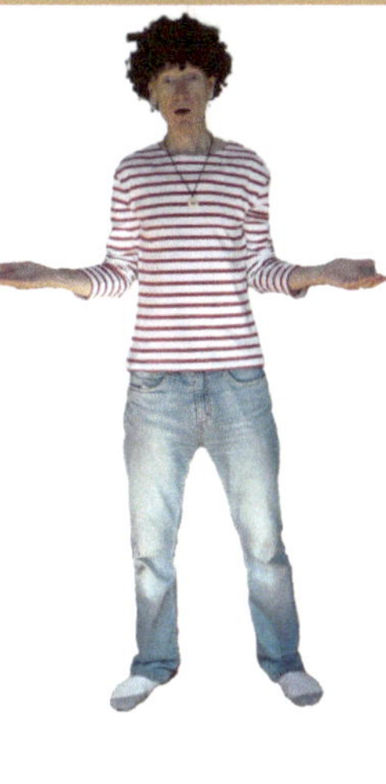

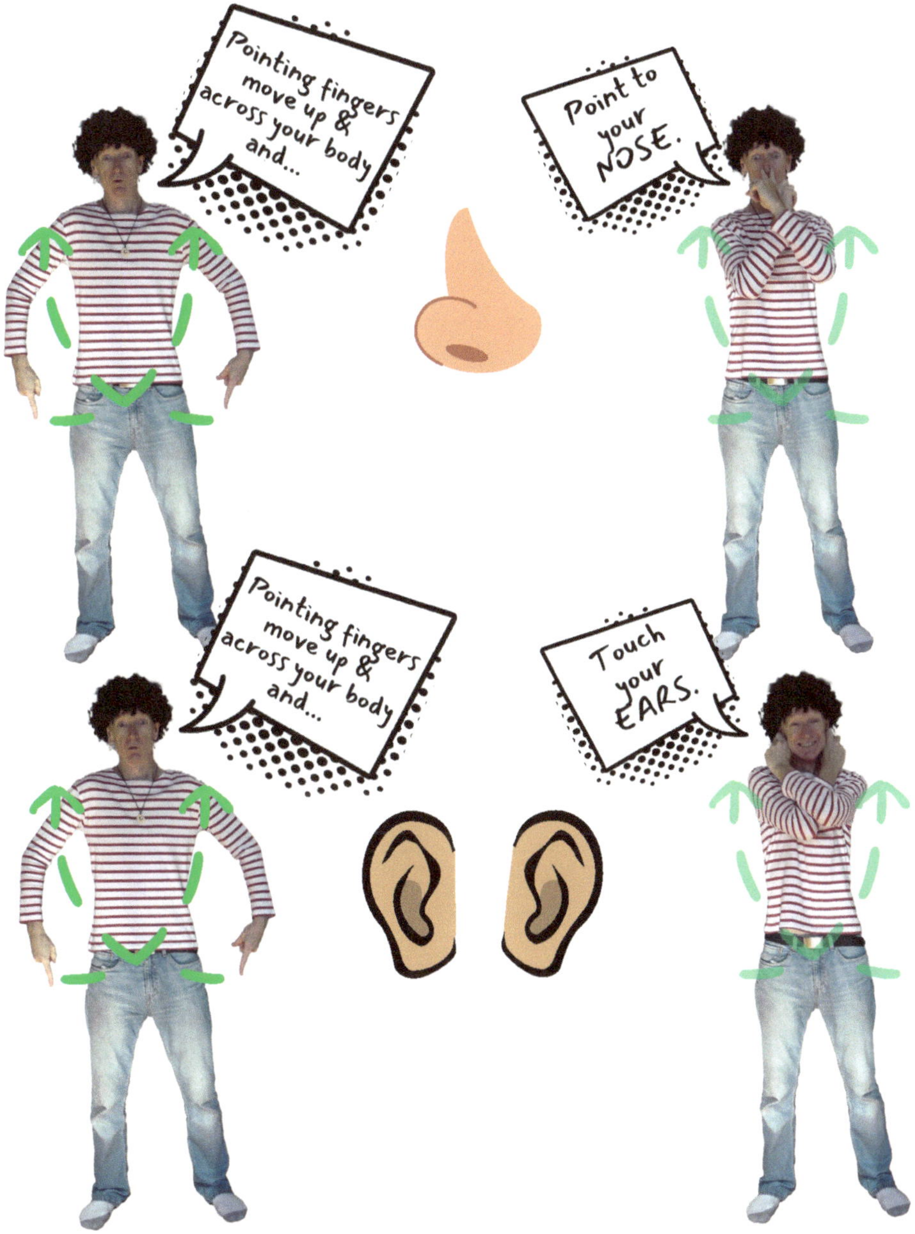

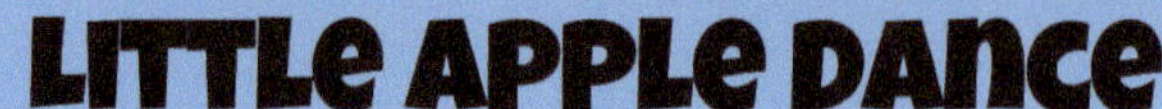

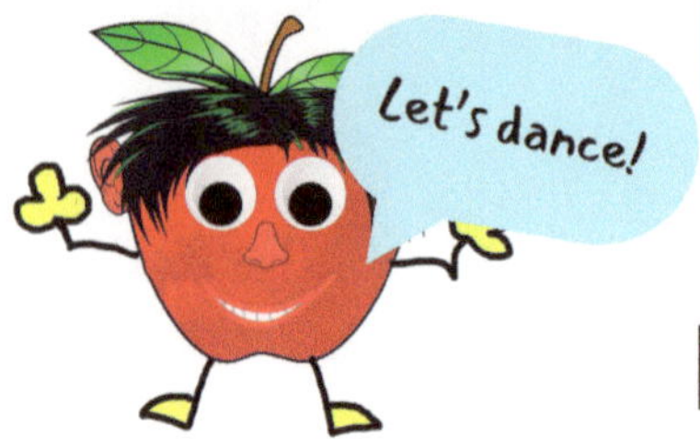

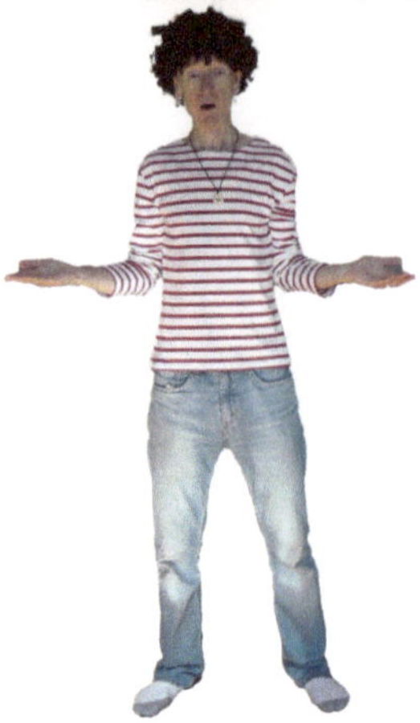

Movement 3
POINT TO BODY PARTS

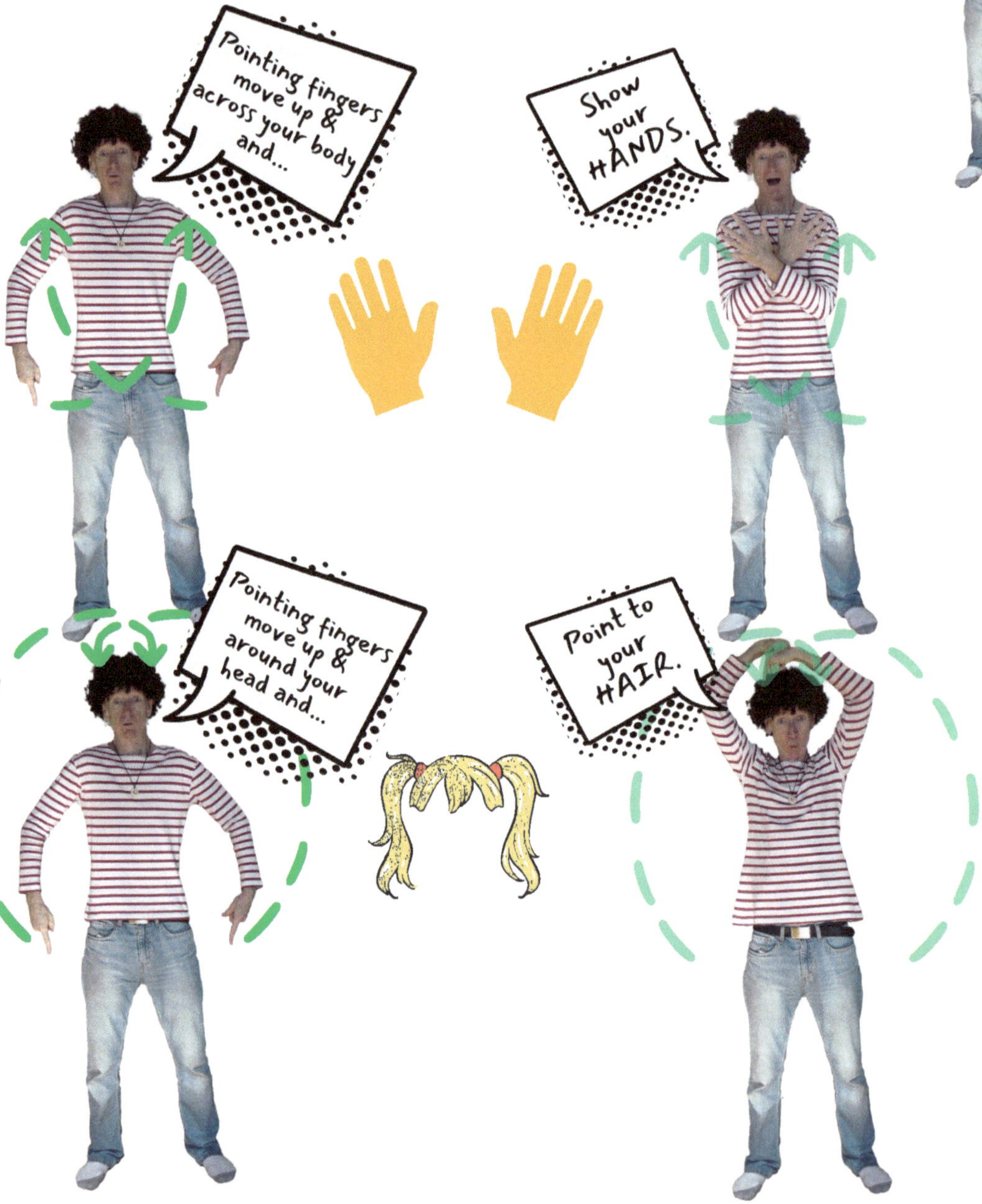

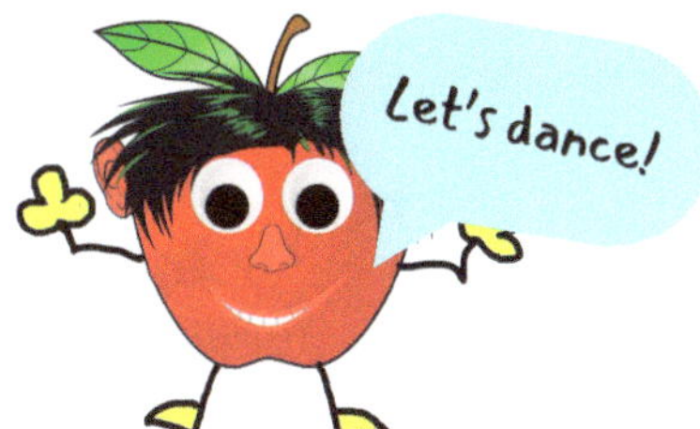

LITTLE APPLE DANCE

Movement 4
CLAPS

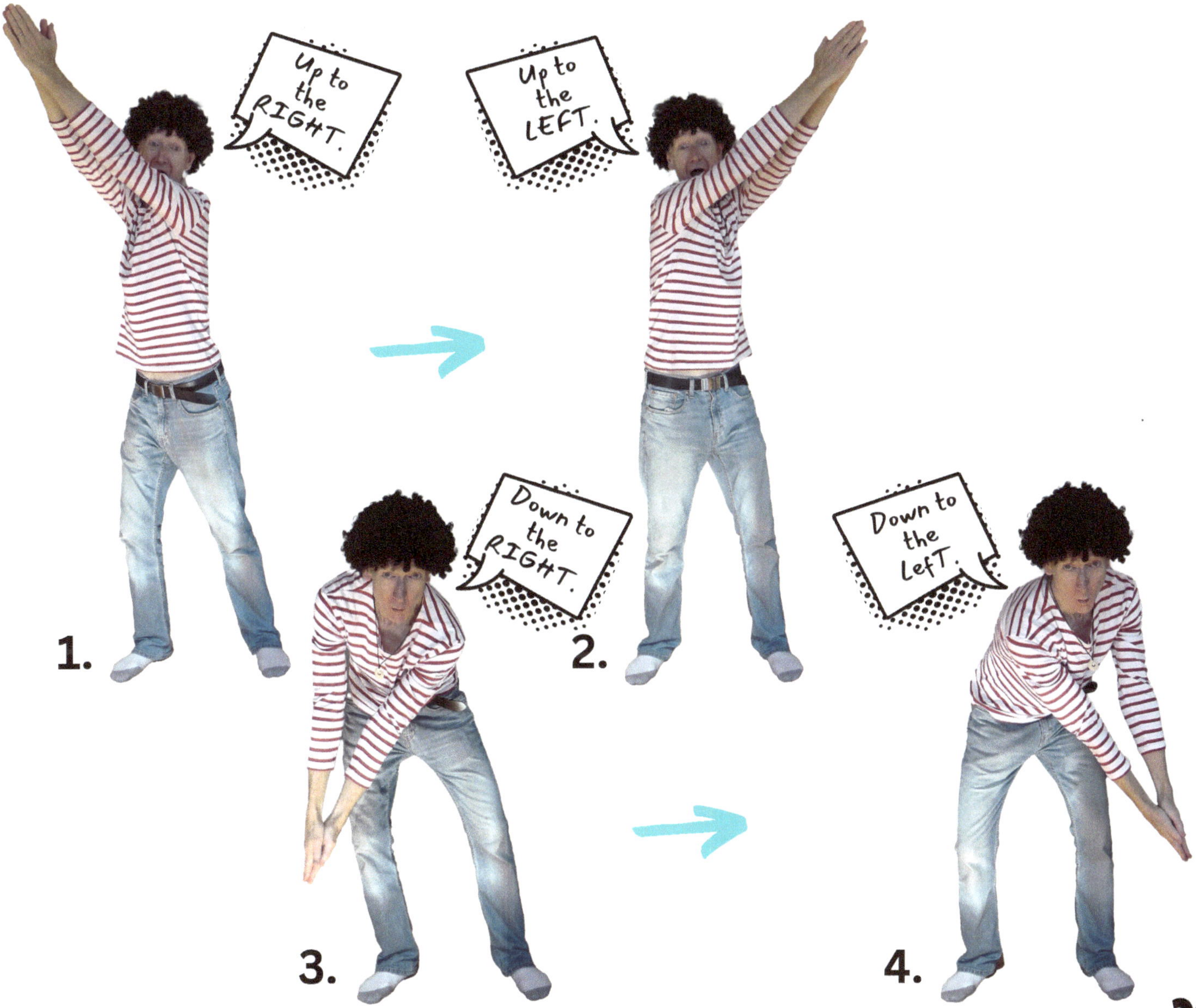

1.

2.

3.

4.

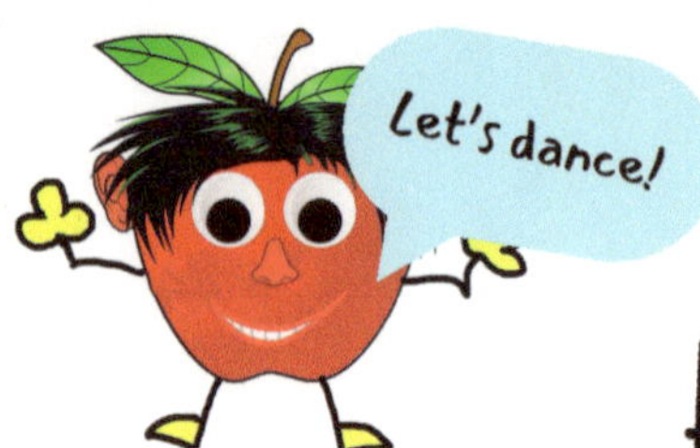

Movement 5
LAZY 8's

Trace an imaginary, sleeping figure of 8 with your hand.

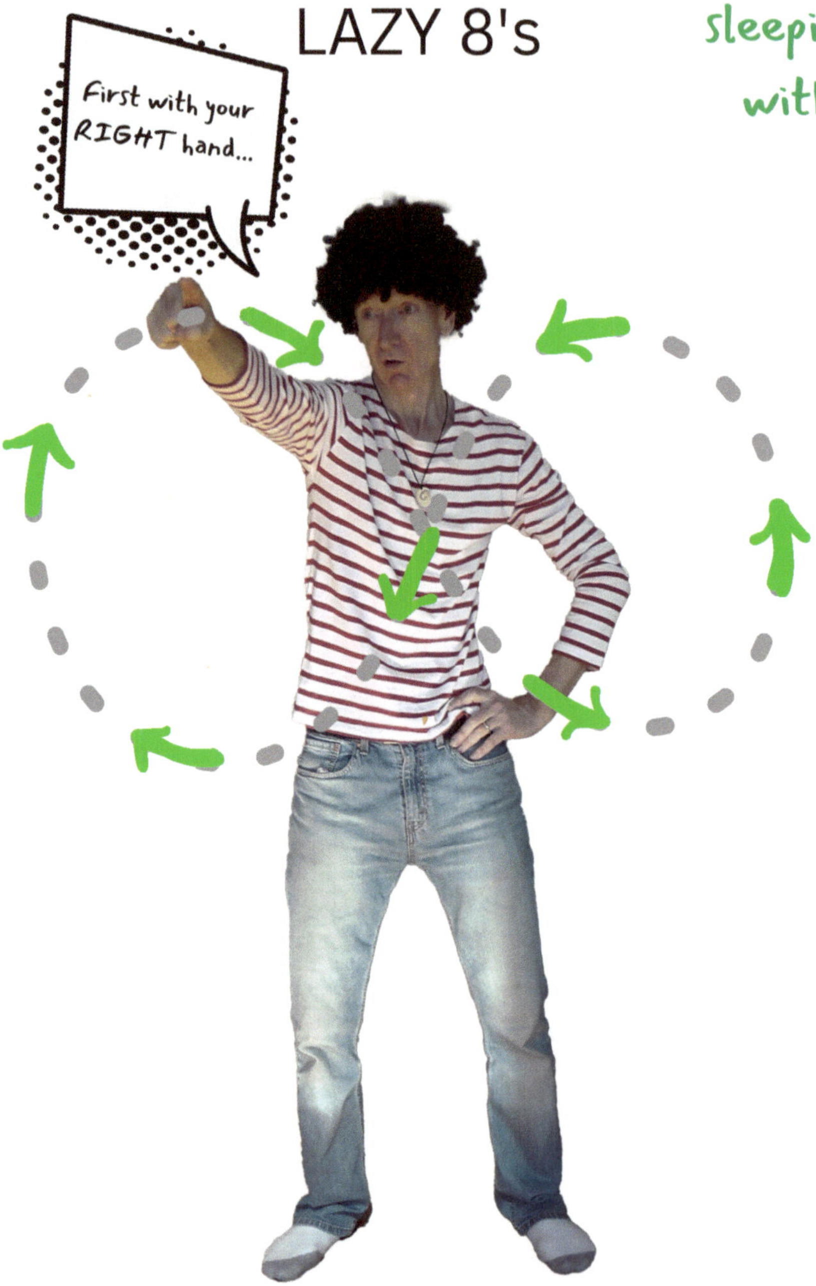

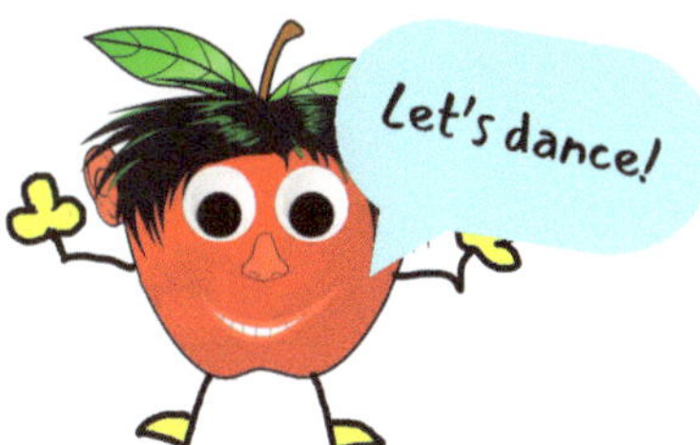

LITTLE APPLE DANCE

Movement 5
LAZY 8's

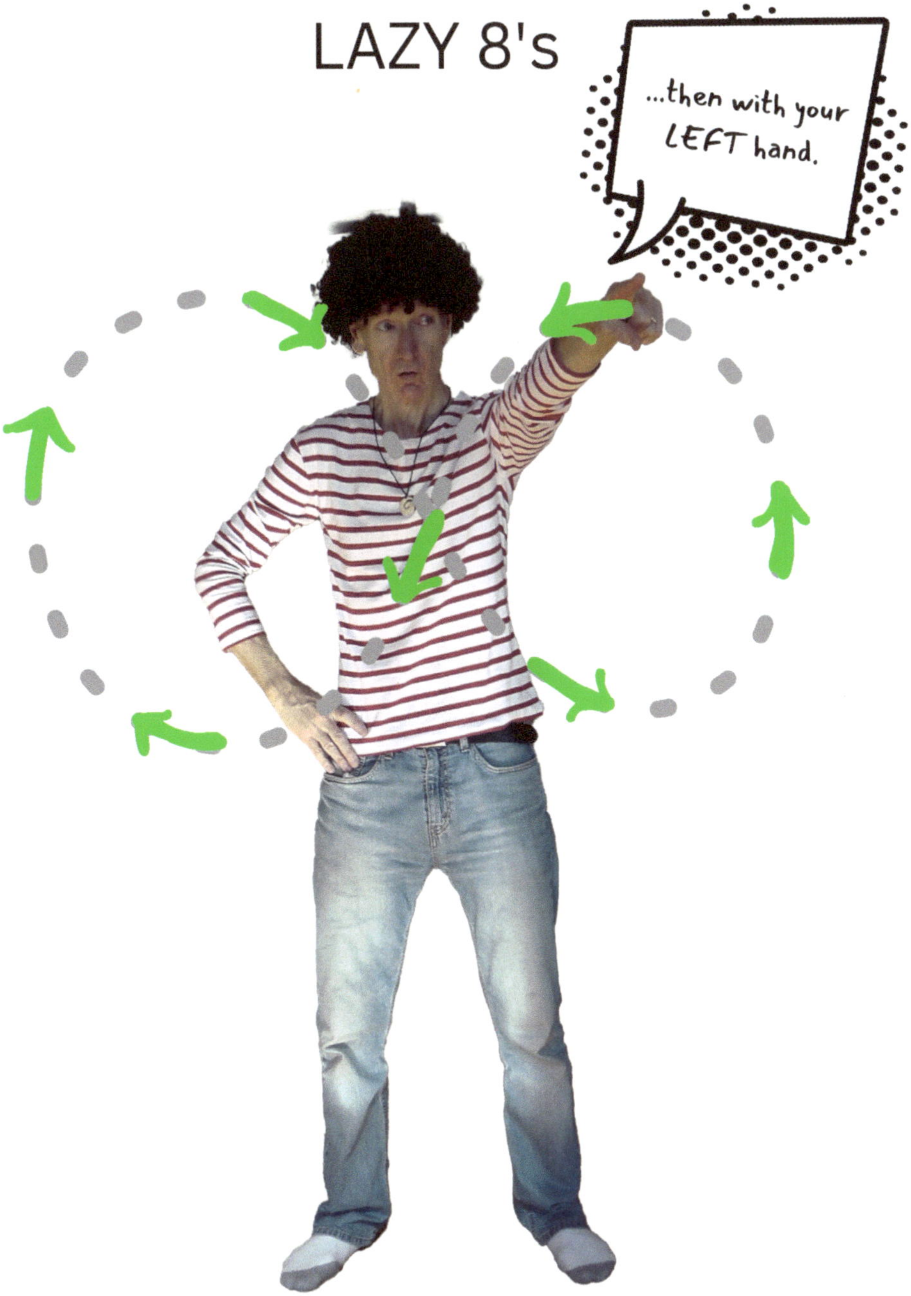

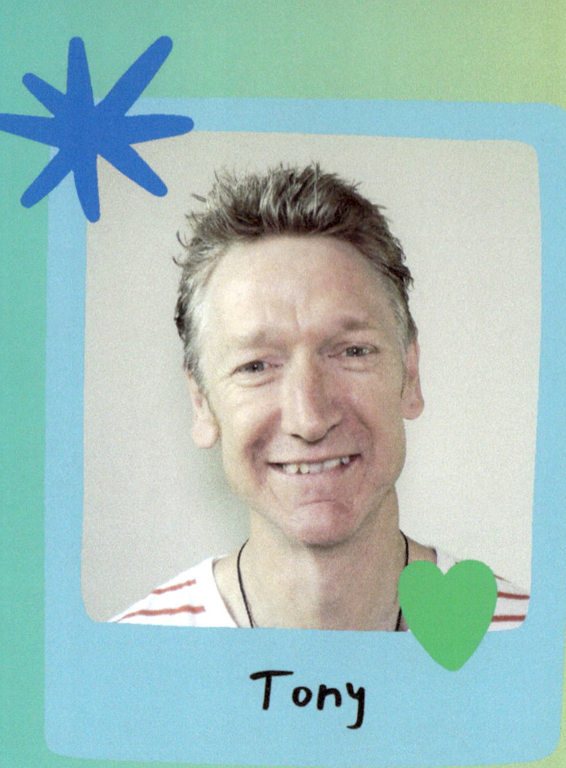

DANCE 3

All right! That was brilliant!

The next dance we're going to learn is with my friend
Little Pear.

Little Pear thinks he is a hip-hop superstar. He sings a
song about numbers. Can you count to ten with him?

There's a photo of Little Pear on the next page...

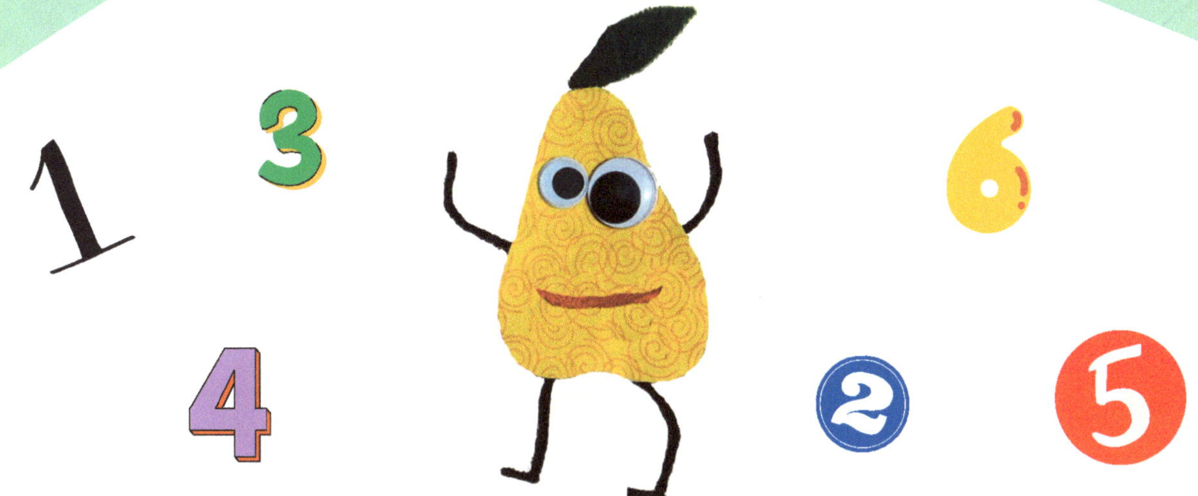

Little Pear LOVES numbers!
And he says it's his birthday...

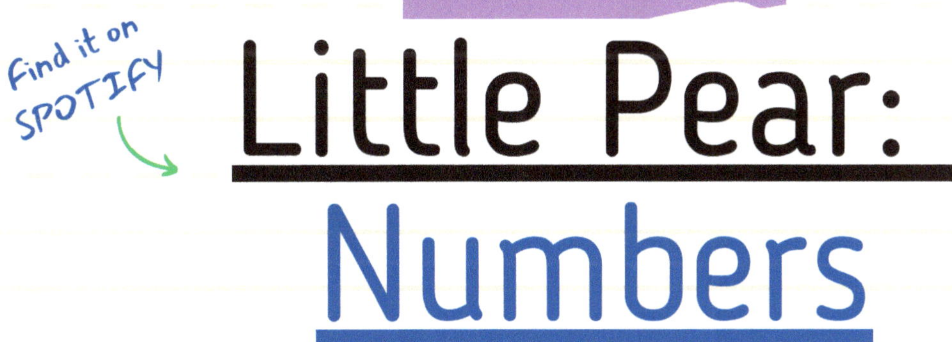

Little Pear: Numbers

Little Pear: Numbers

Happy Birthday to you, Little Pear. *(repeat)*
How old are you, Little Pear? *(repeat)* } CHORUS

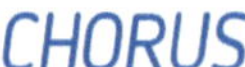

I'm 3... 3! Yeah I'm 3... 3!
1, 2, 3. Yeah!
(3, 2, 1, Go!)

CHORUS

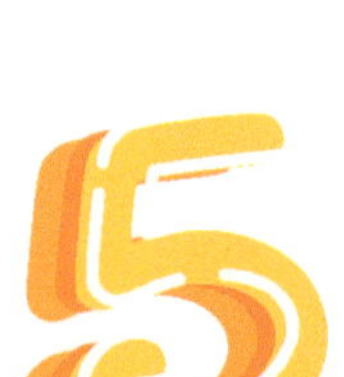

I'm 5... 5! Yeah I'm 5... 5!
1, 2, 3, 4, 5. Yeah!
(5, 4, 3, 2, 1, Go!)

CHORUS

I'm 7... 7! Yeah I'm 7... 7!
1, 2, 3, 4, 5, 6, 7. Yeah!
(7, 6, 5, 4, 3, 2, 1, Go!)

CHORUS

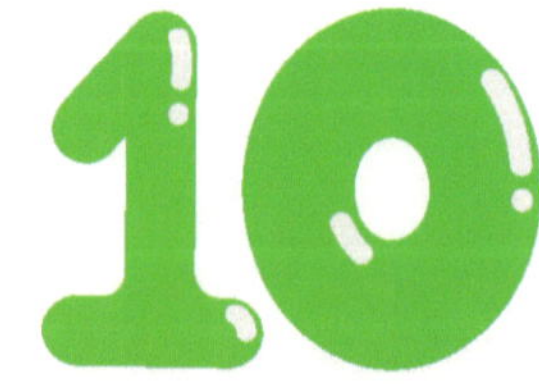

I'm 10... 10! Yeah I'm 10... 10!
1, 2, 3, 4, 5, 6, 7, 8, 9... 10. Yeah!
(10, 9, 8, 7, 6, 5, 4, 3, 2, 1, Go!)

LITTLE PEAR DANCE

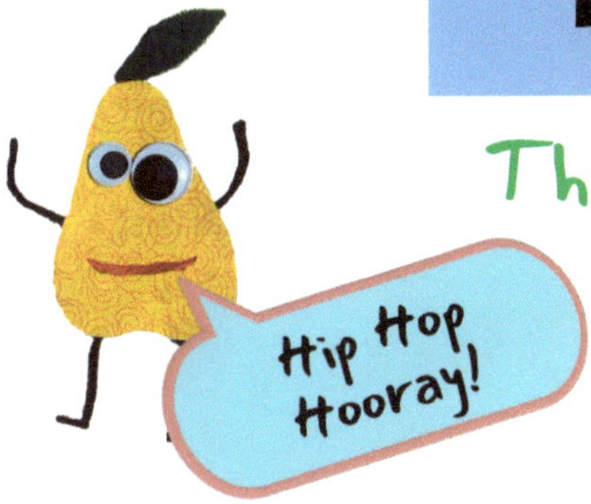

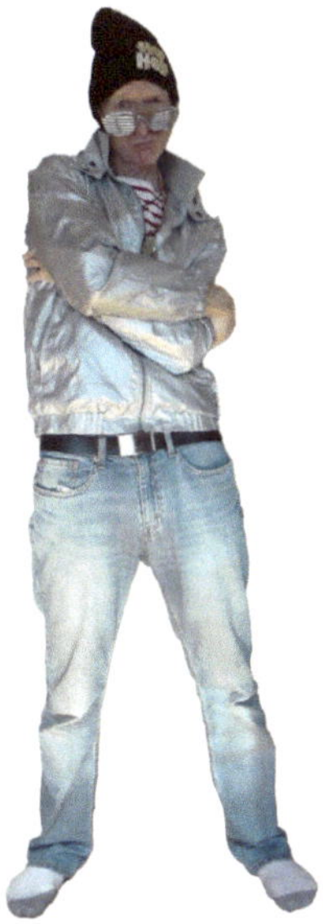

This dance involves 3 movements.

Movement 1
Cross Crawl

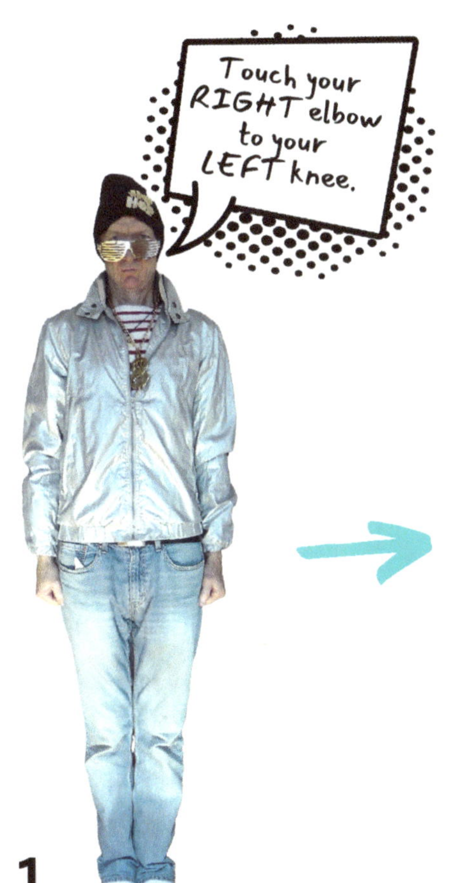

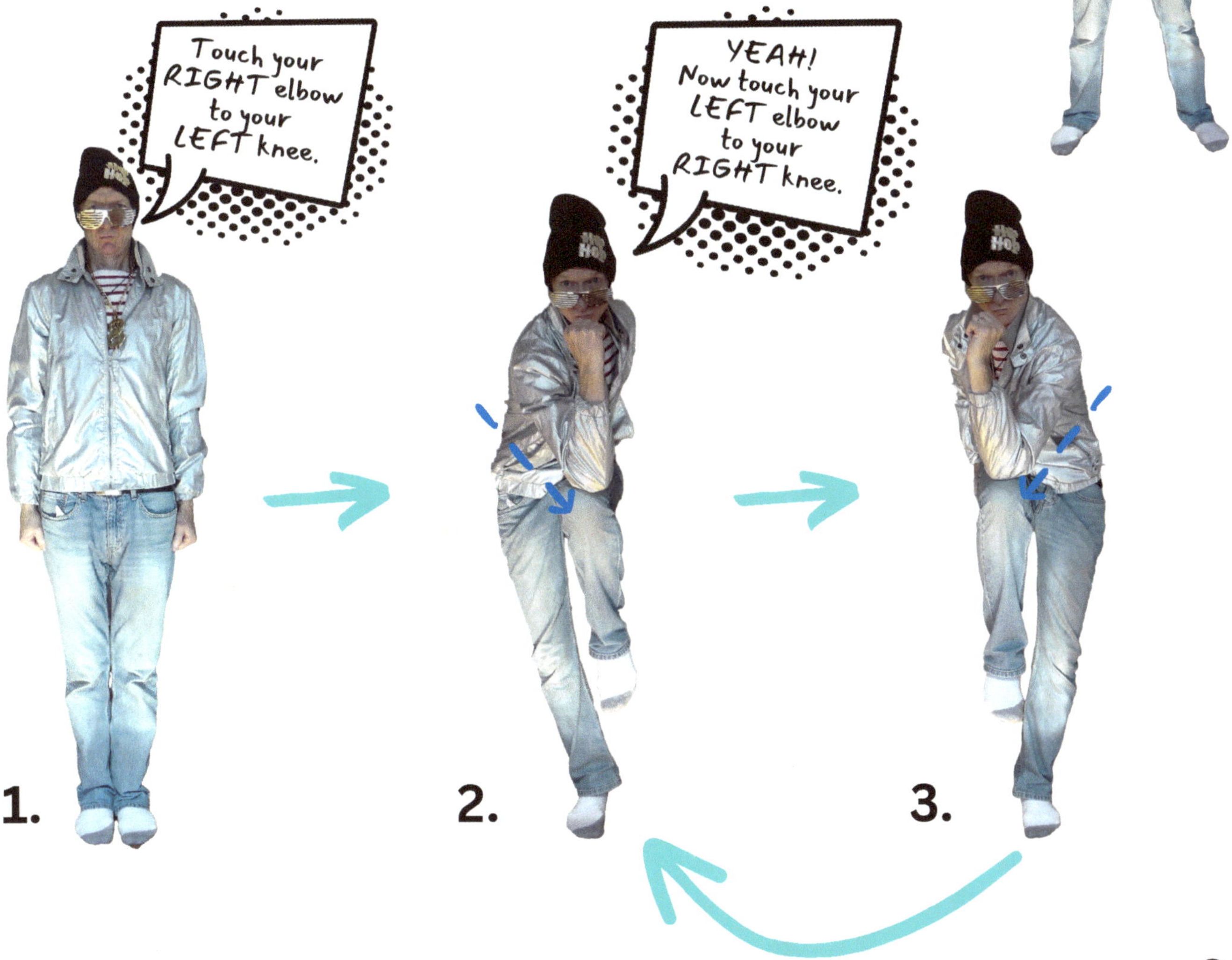

LITTLE PEAR DANCE

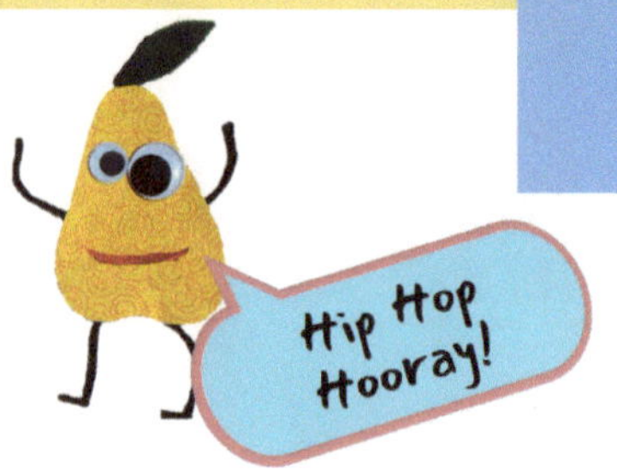

Movement 2
Drive the car

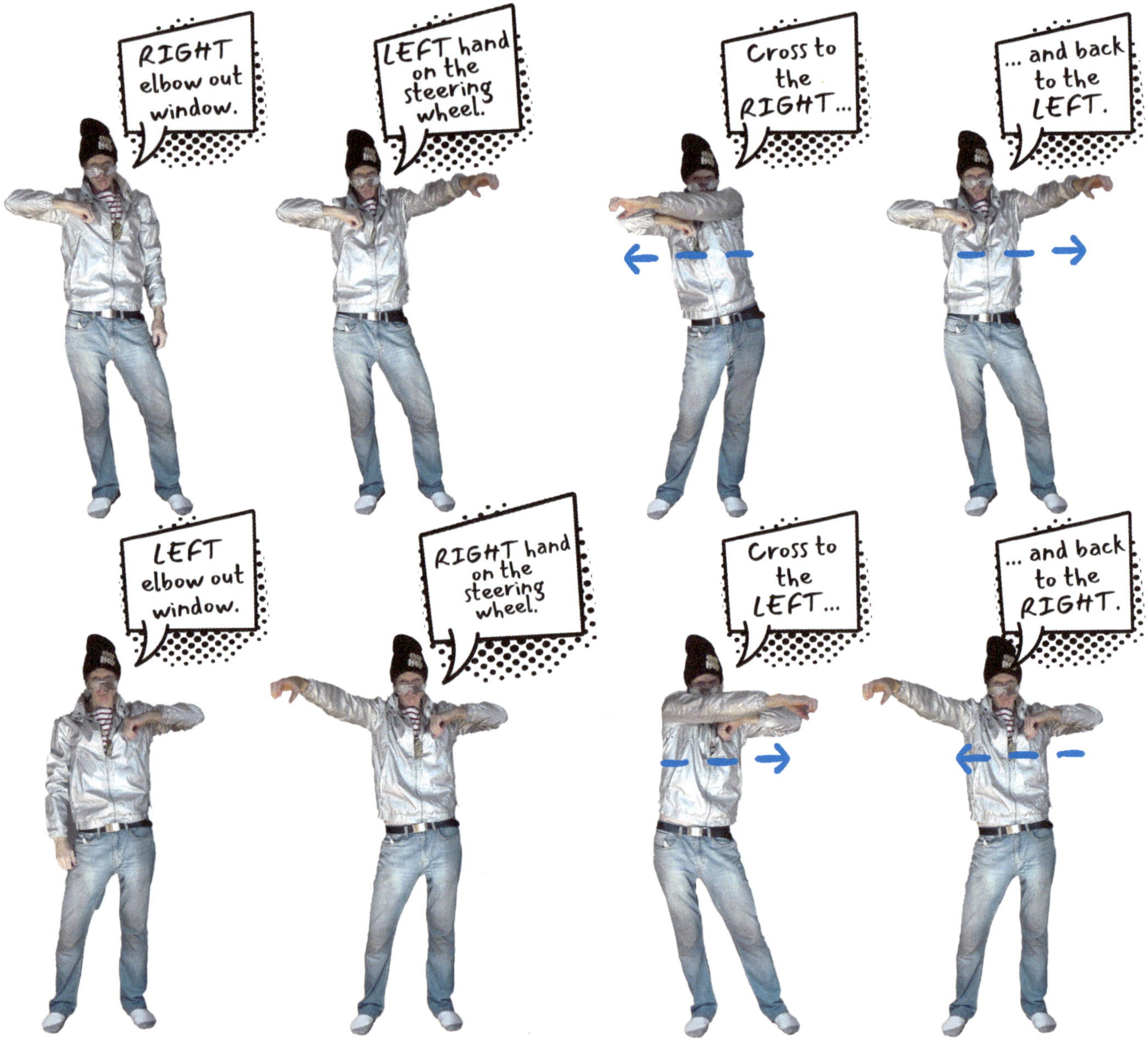

LITTLE PEAR DANCE

Movement 3
Counting
Jump & Cross

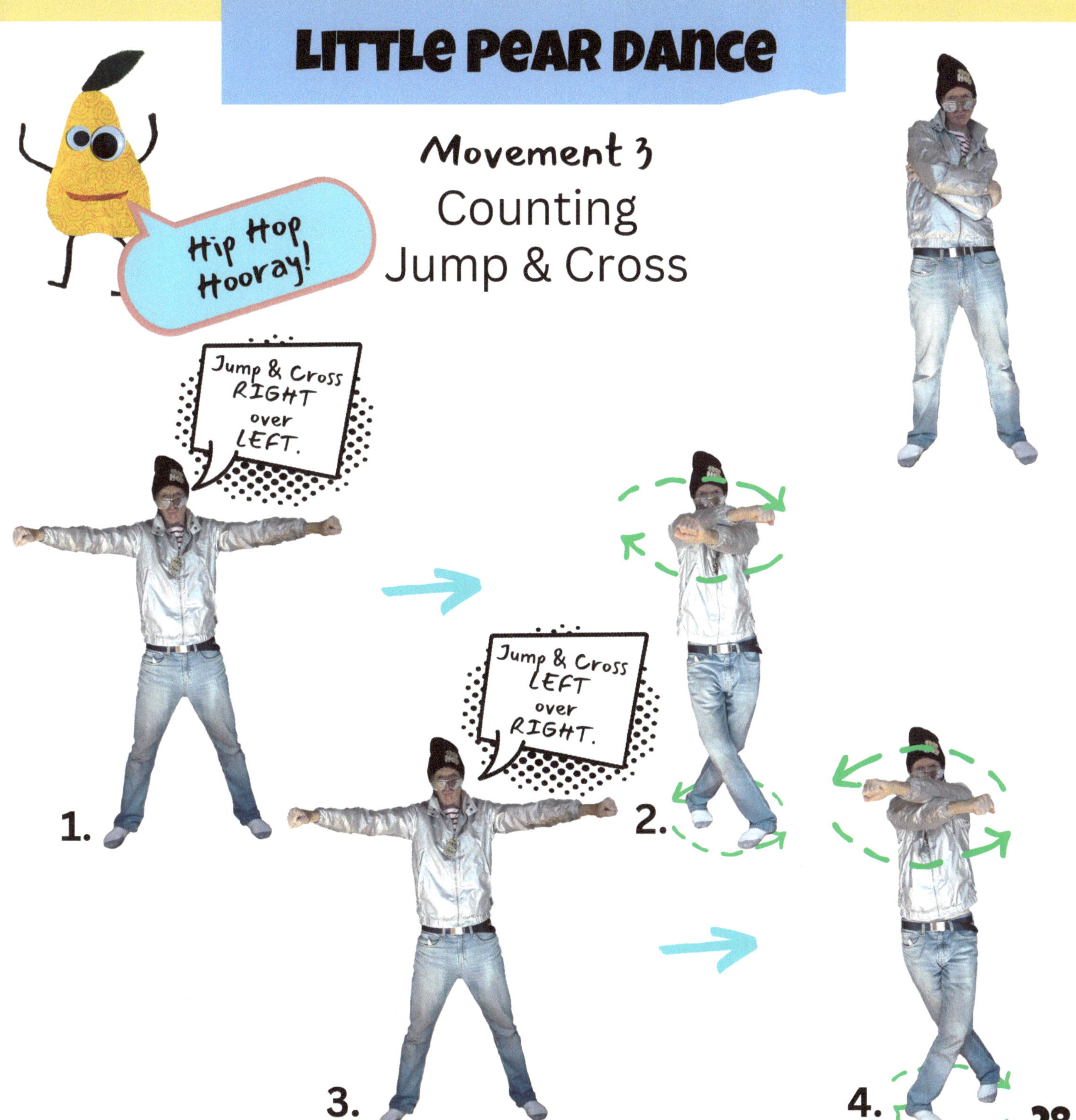

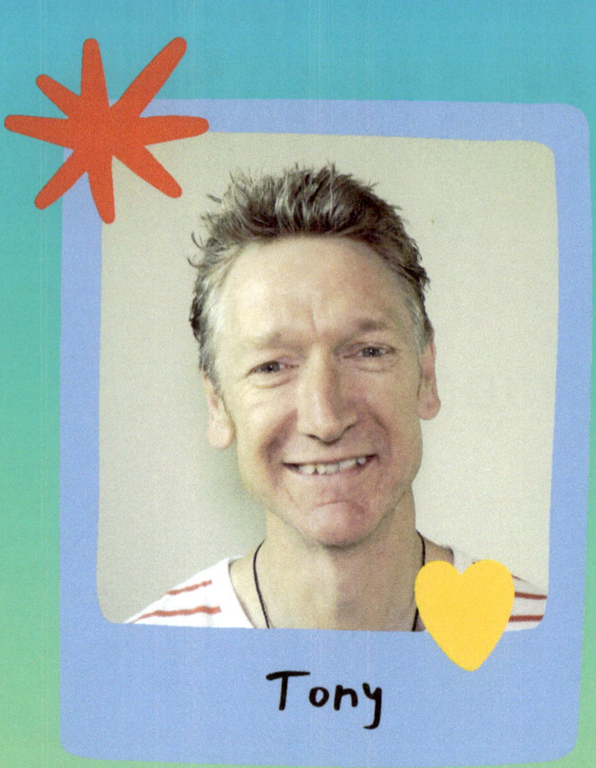

DANCE 4

Yippee! That was awesome!

The next dance we're going to learn is with my friend **Little Potato.**

Little Potato sings a song about sports. Do you like sports? What is your favourite sport?

There's a photo of Little Potato on the next page...

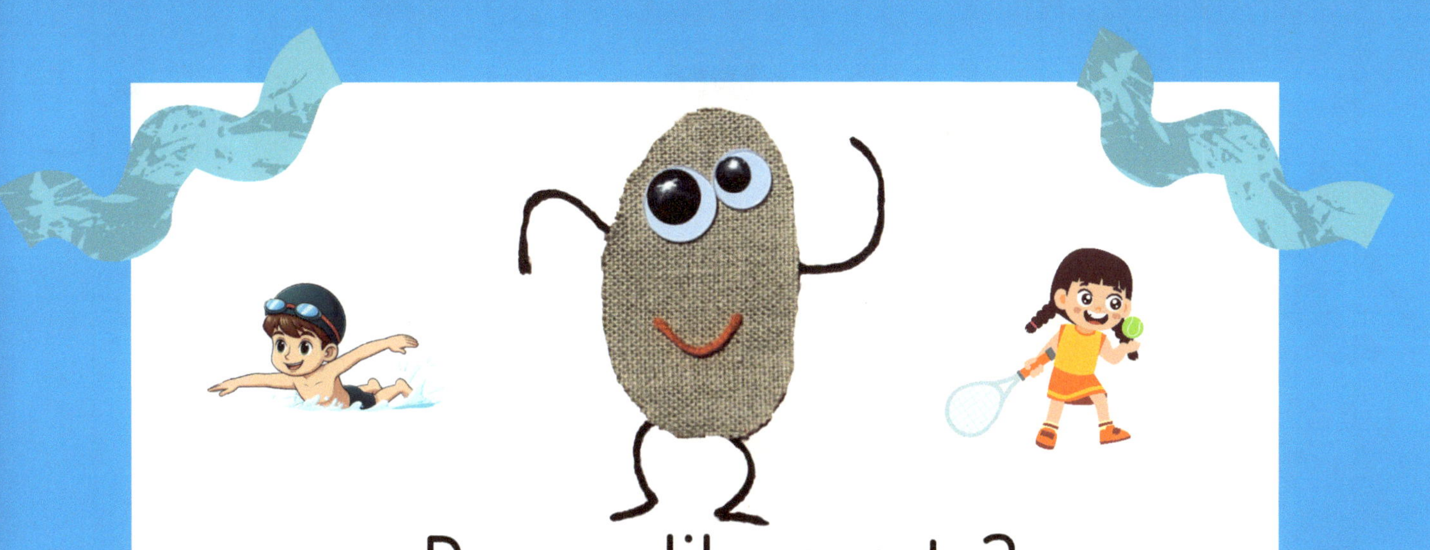

Do you like sports?
Little Potato wants to play!

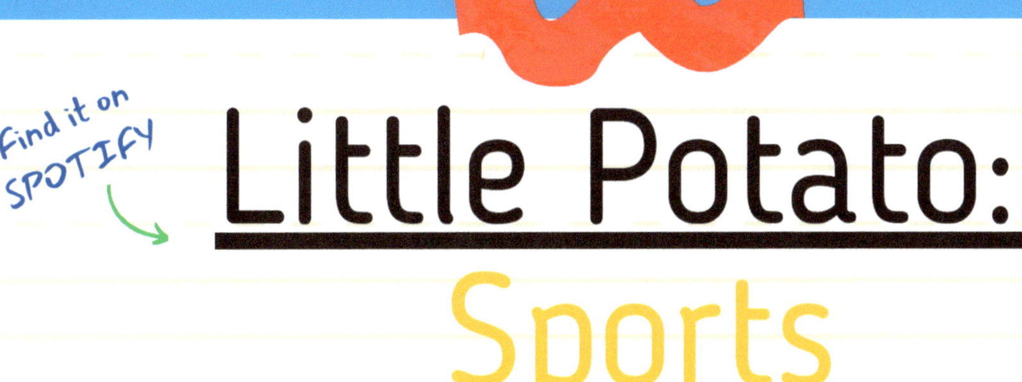

Little Potato:

Sports

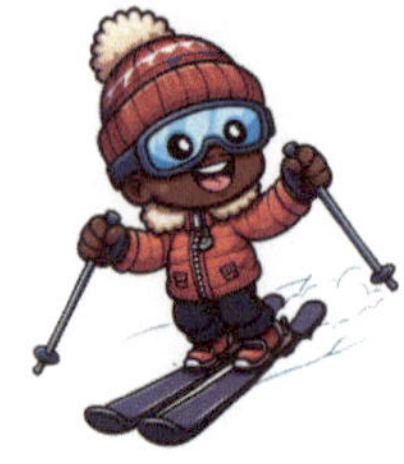
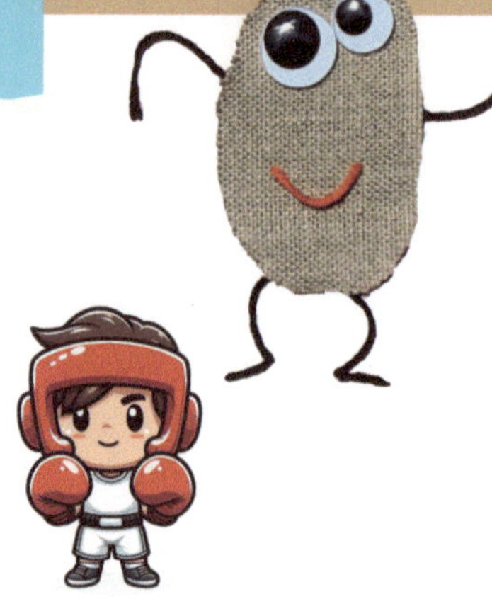

Little Potato, ready, steady, go. Do you like skiing?
Yes I like skiing!

Little Potato, ready, steady, go. Do you like boxing?
Yes I like boxing!

Little Potato, ready, steady, go. Do you like swimming?
Yes I like swimming!

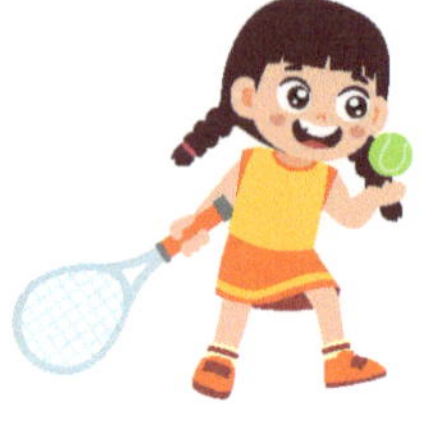

Little Potato, go, go, go. *(repeat)*

Little Potato, ready, steady, go. Do you like dancing?
Yes I like dancing!

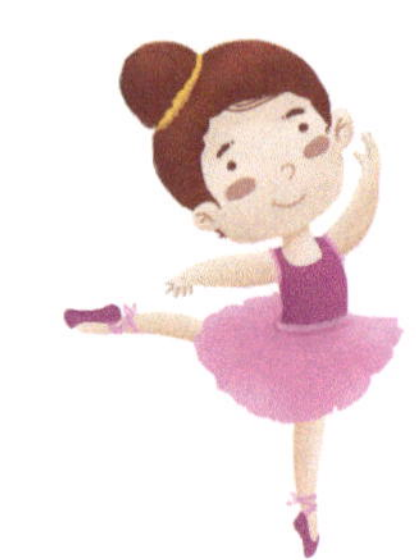

Little Potato, ready, steady, go. Do you like tennis?
Yes I like tennis!

Little Potato, ready, steady, go. Do you like rugby?
Yes I like rugby!
Do you like tennis? Yes I like tennis!
Do you like dancing? Yes I like dancing!
Do you like swimming? Yes I like swimming!
Do you like boxing? Yes I like boxing!
Do you like skiing? Yes I like skiing!

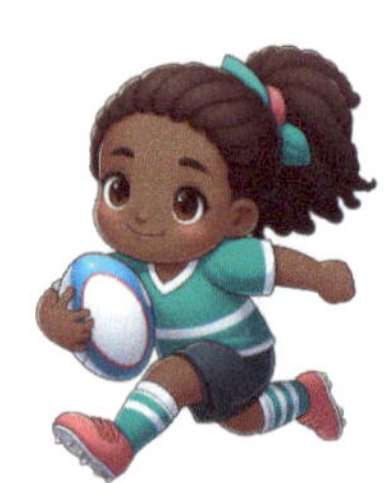
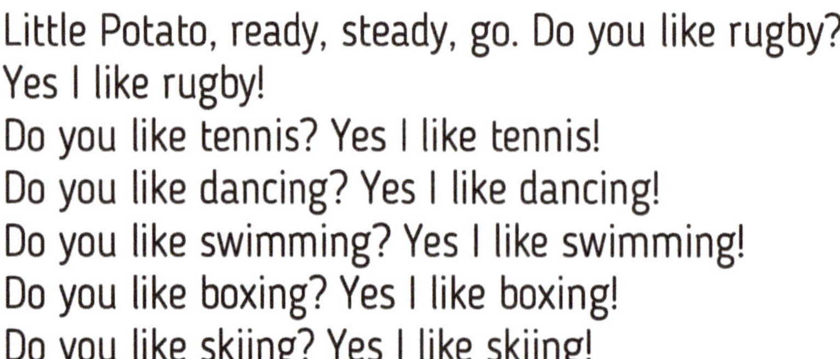

Little Potato, go, go, go. *(repeat x 4)*

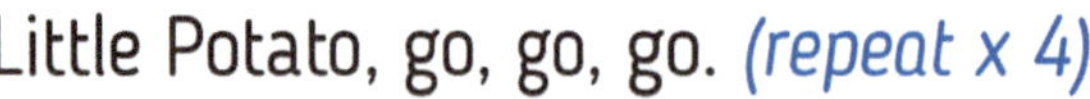

LITTLE POTATO DANCE

This dance involves 8 movements.

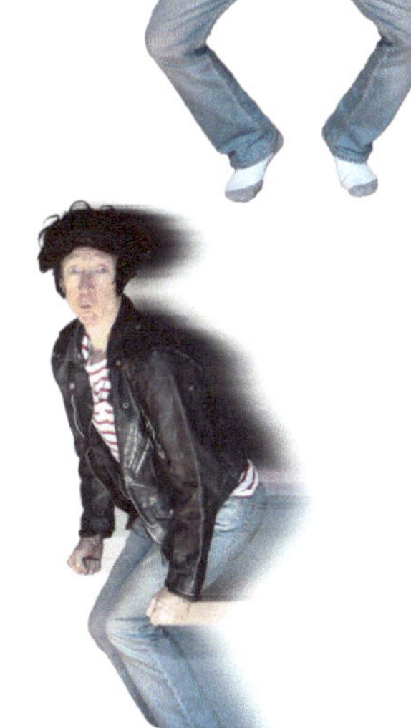

Movement 1
Skiing

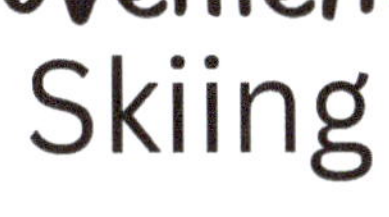

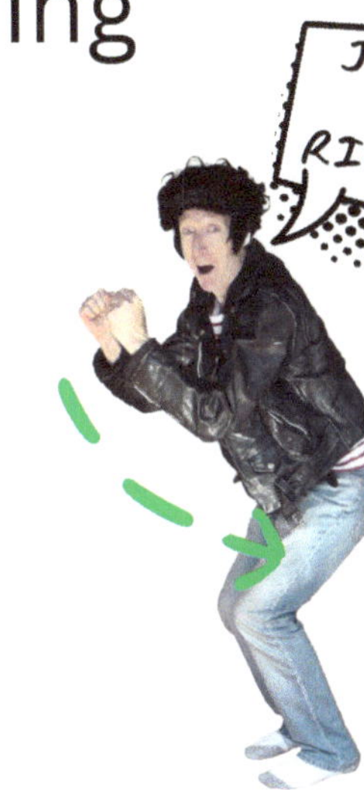

Movement 2
Boxing

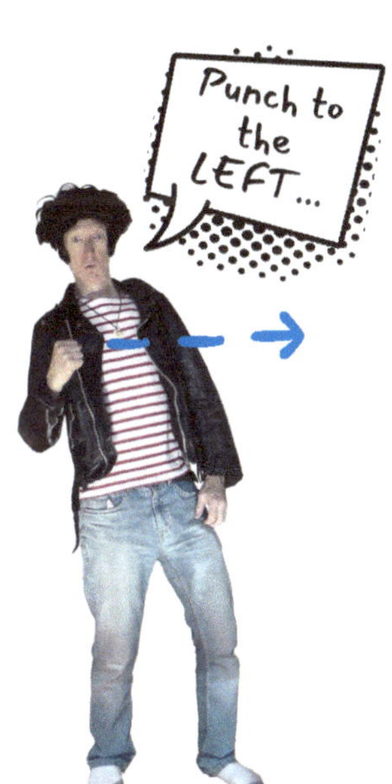

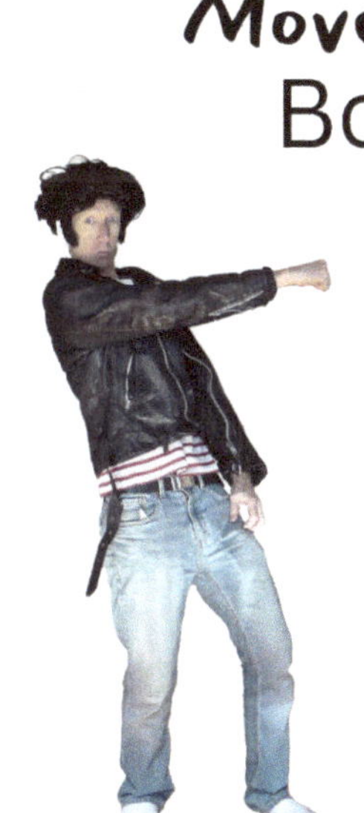

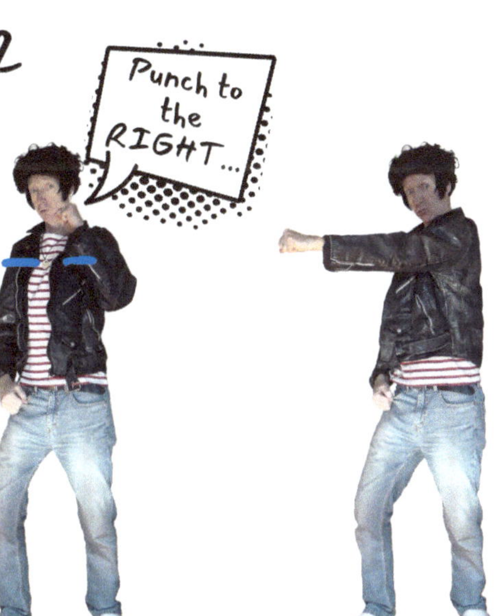

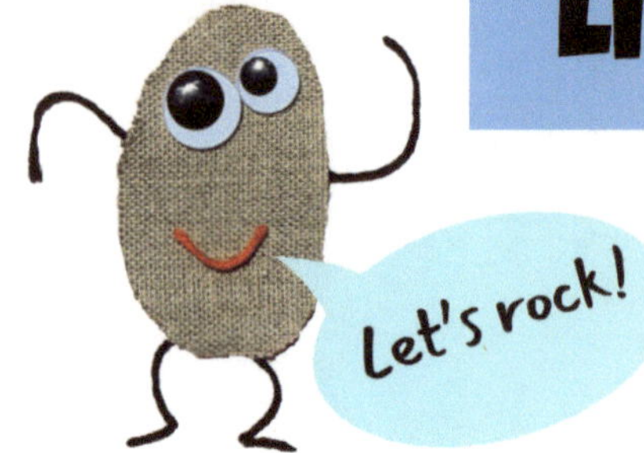

Movement 3
Swimming

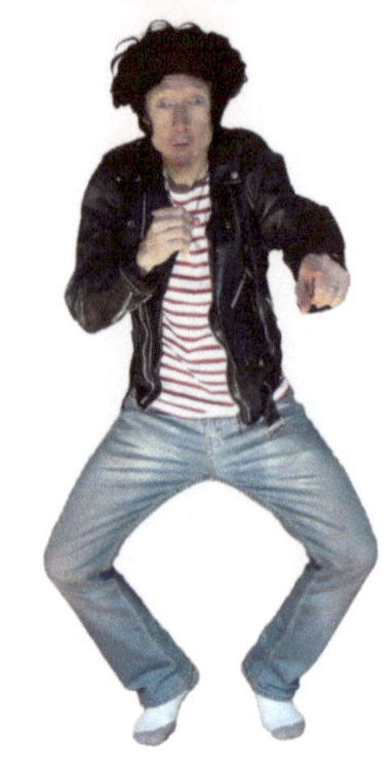

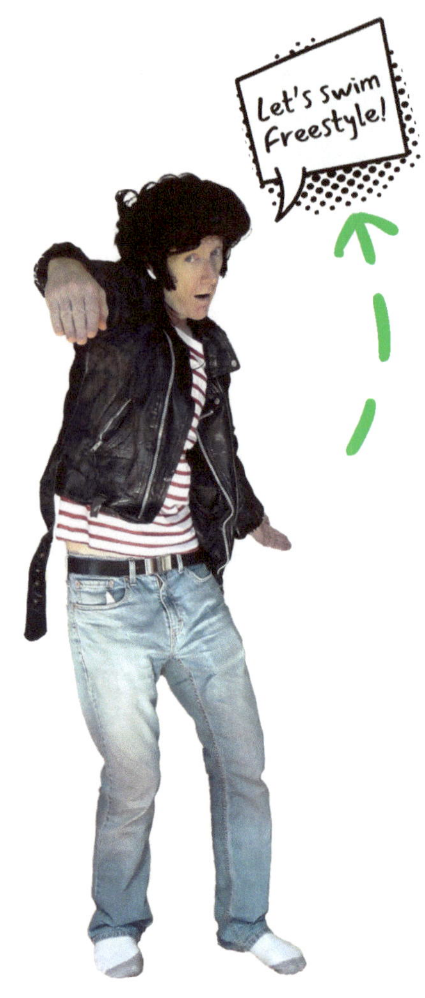

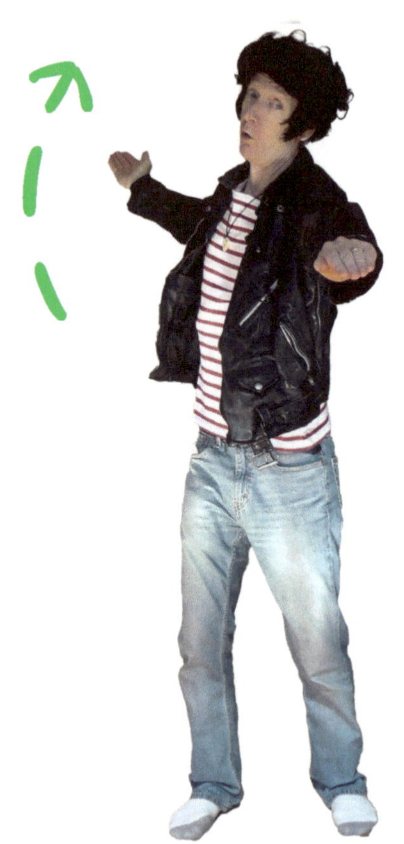

LITTLE POTATO DANCE

Movement 4
Bee's Knees Dance

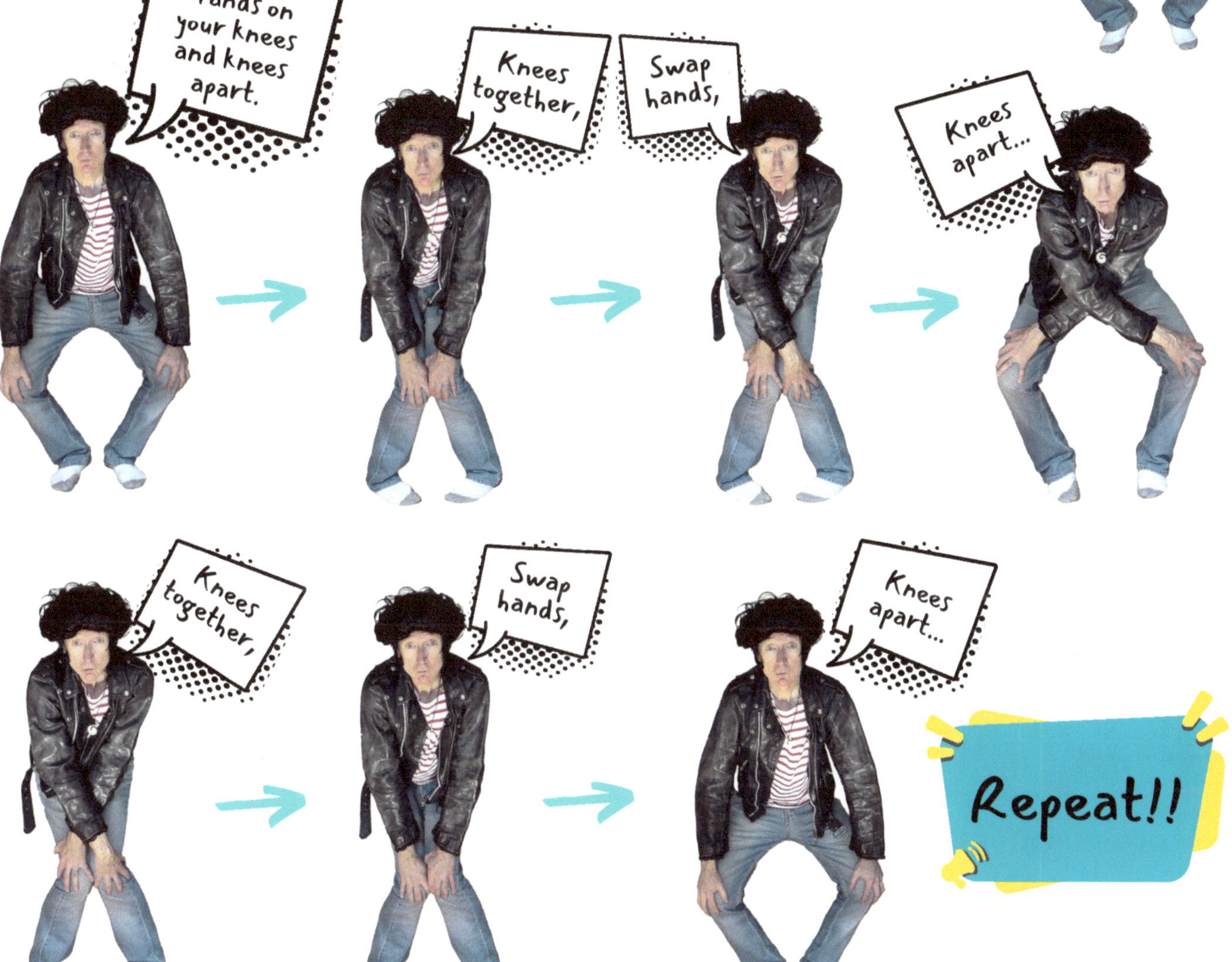

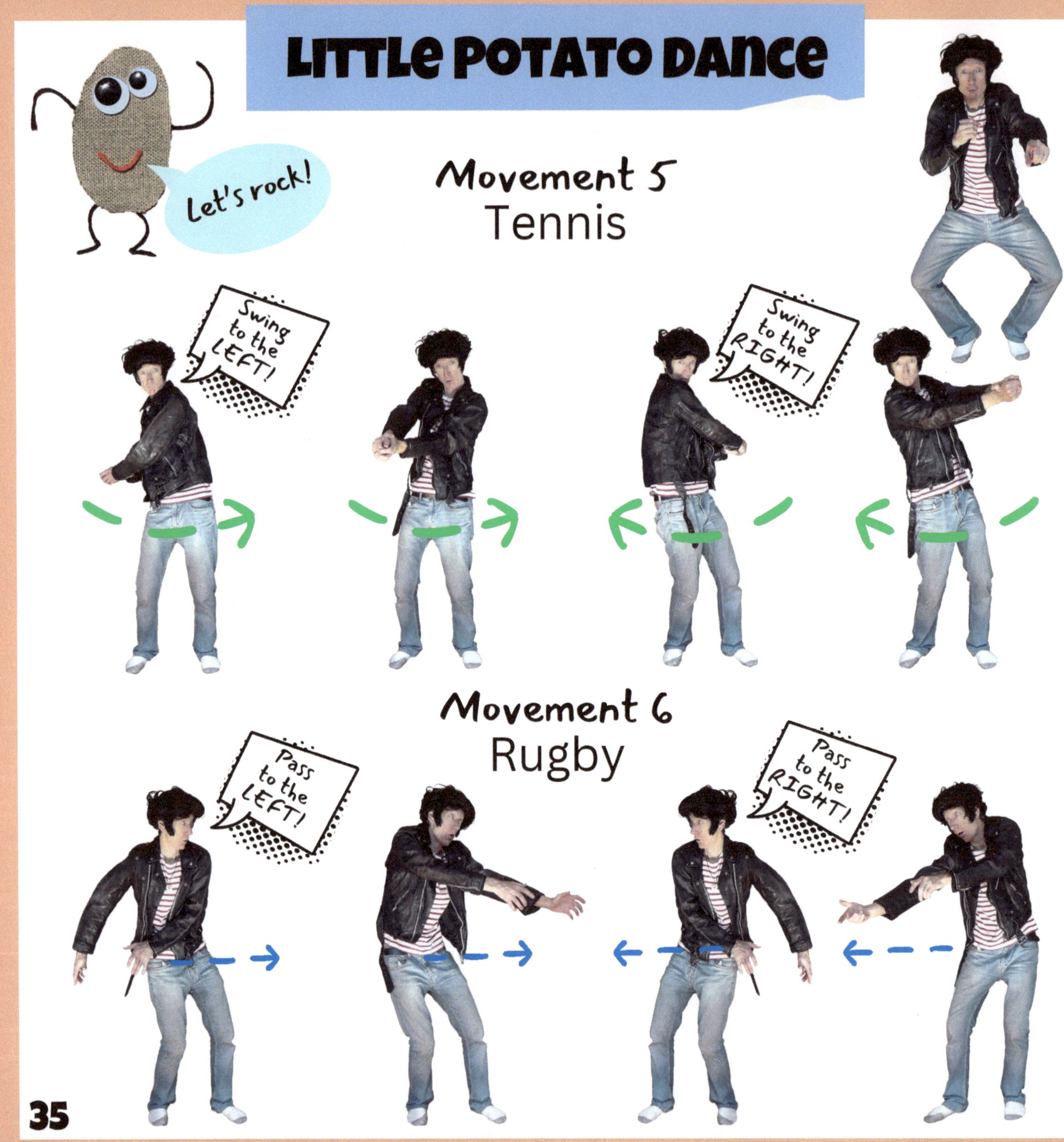

LITTLE POTATO DANCE

Movement 5
Tennis

Movement 6
Rugby

LITTLE POTATO DANCE

Movement 7
The Twist

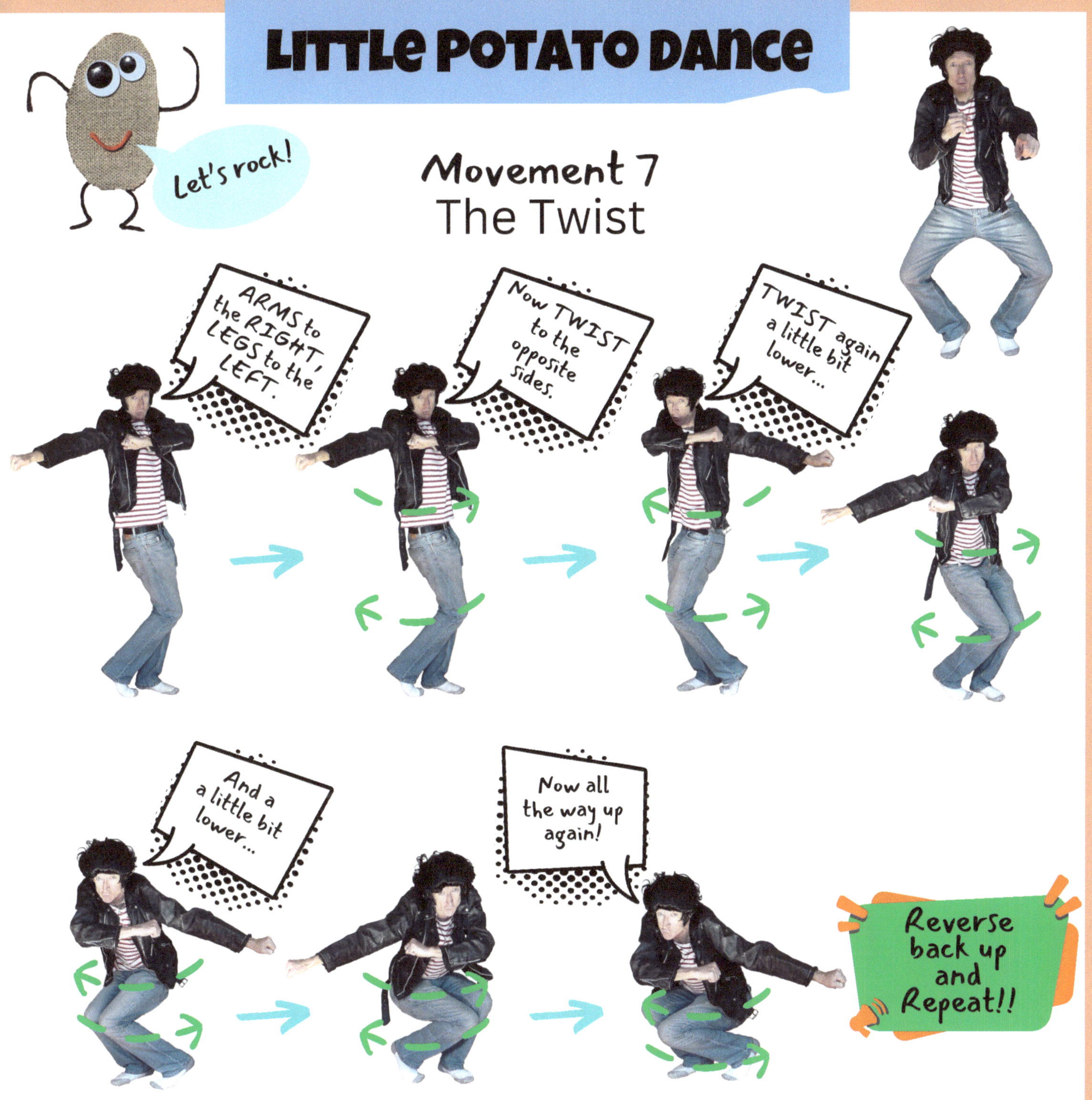

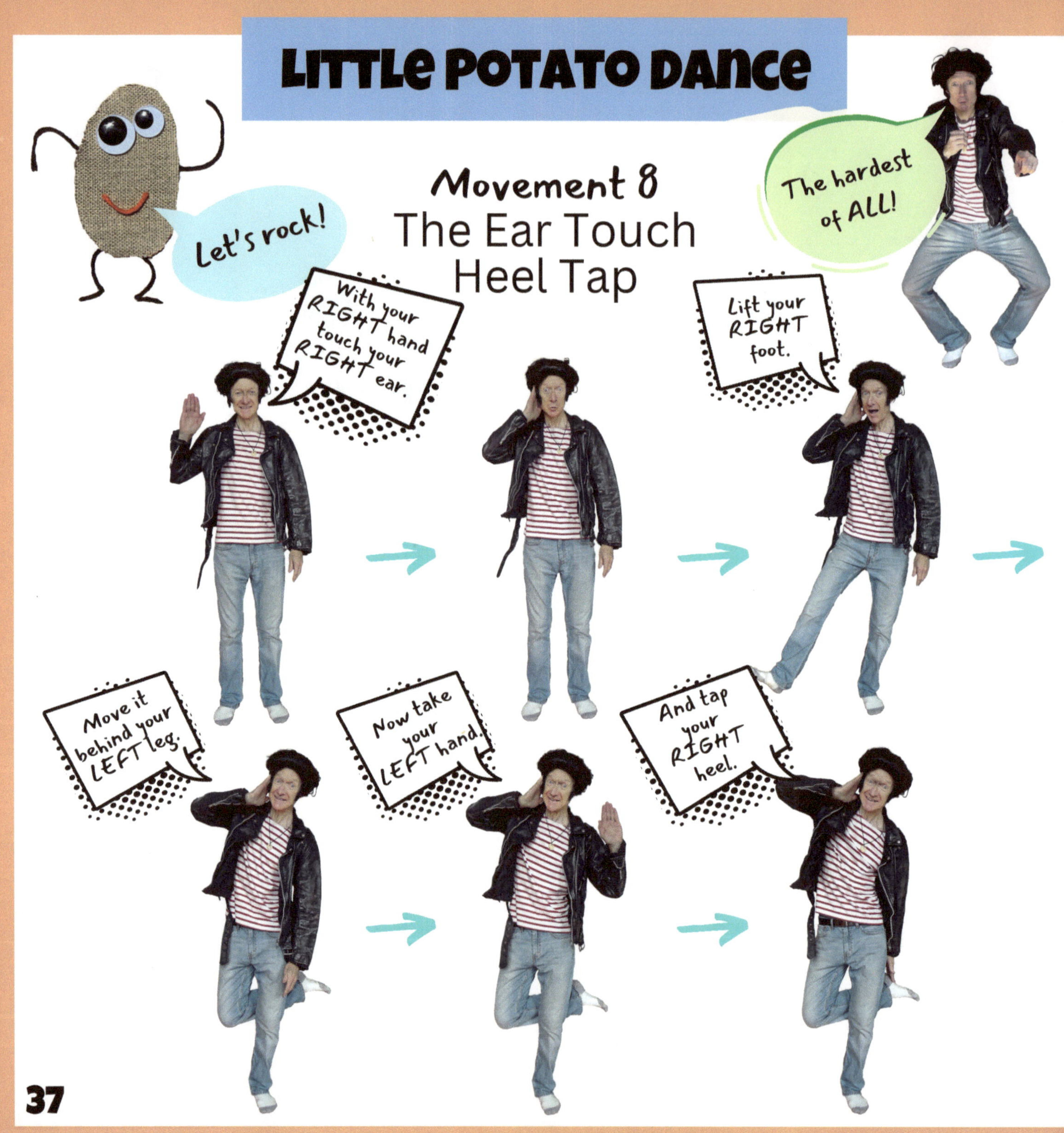

LITTLE POTATO DANCE
Let's rock!
Movement 8
The Ear Touch
Heel Tap
The hardest of ALL!
With your RIGHT hand touch your RIGHT ear.
Lift your RIGHT foot.
Move it behind your LEFT leg.
Now take your LEFT hand.
And tap your RIGHT heel.

LITTLE POTATO DANCE

Movement 8
The Ear Touch Heel Tap

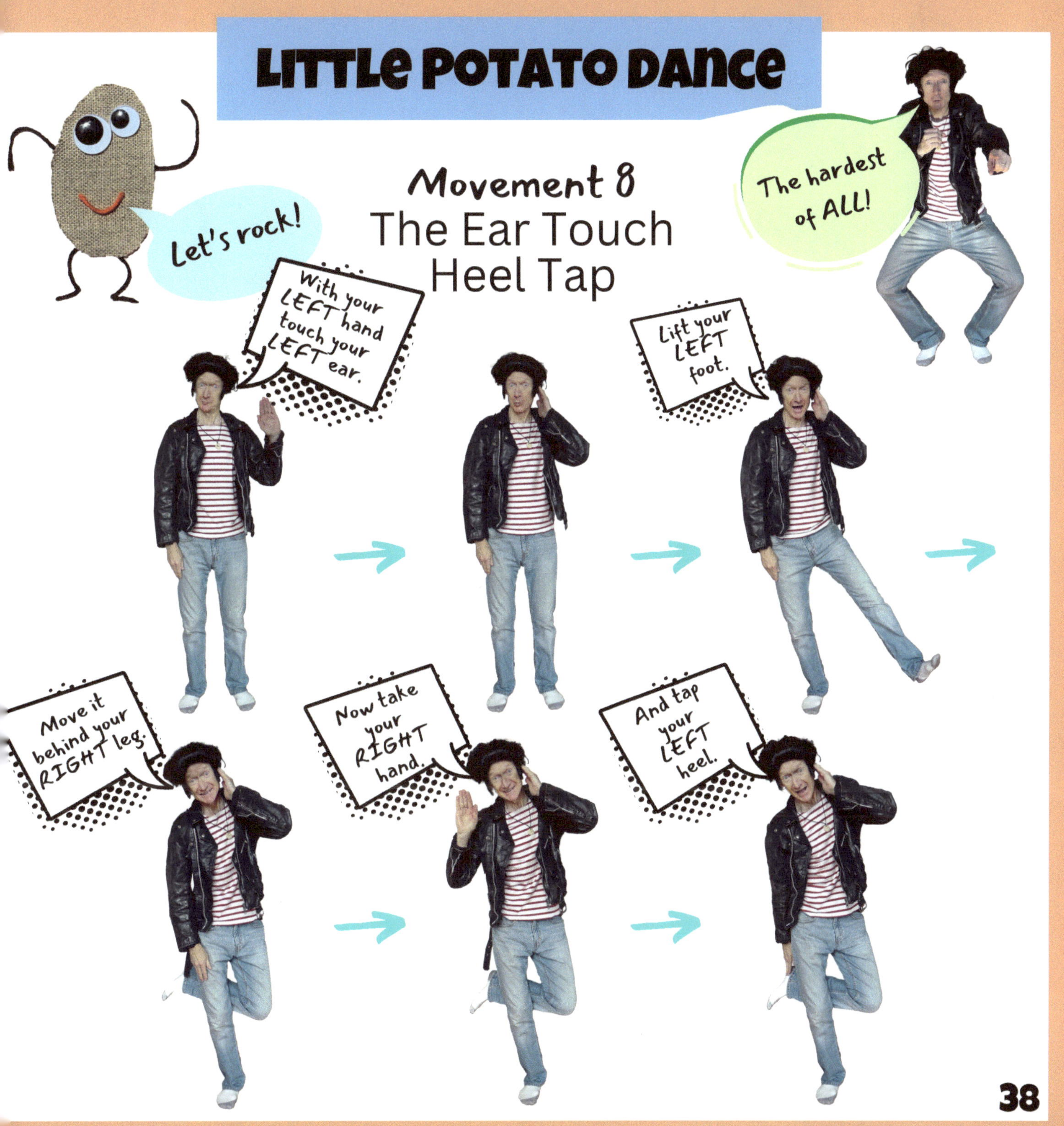

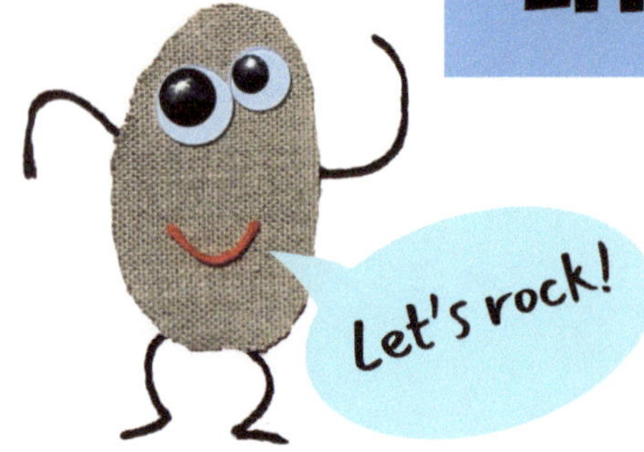

Movement 8
The Ear Touch Heel Tap

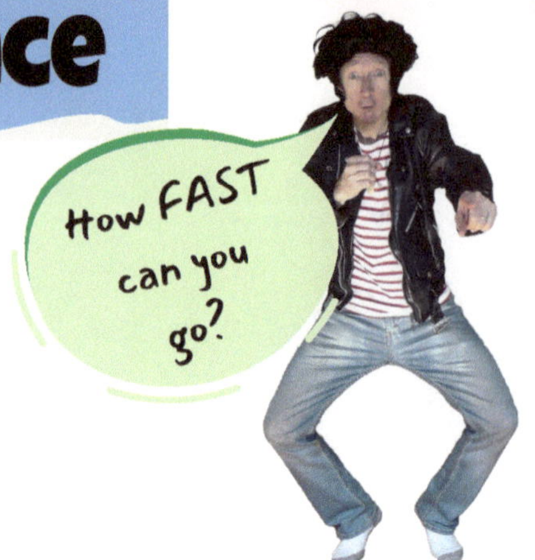

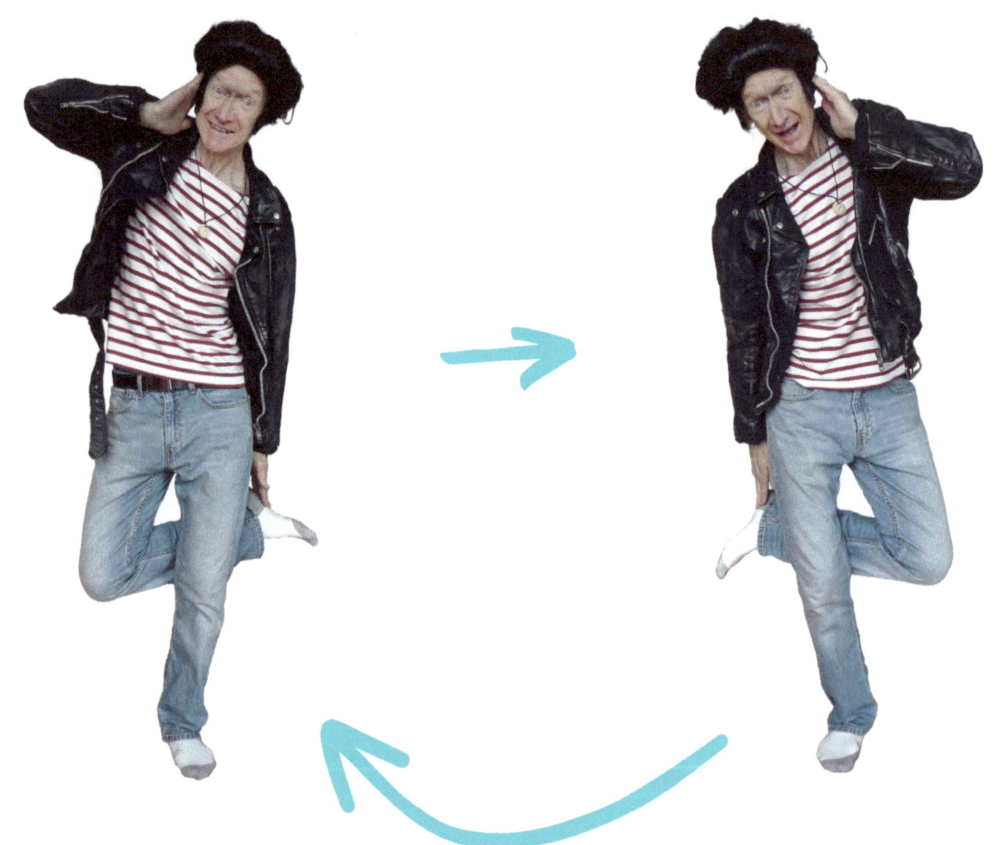

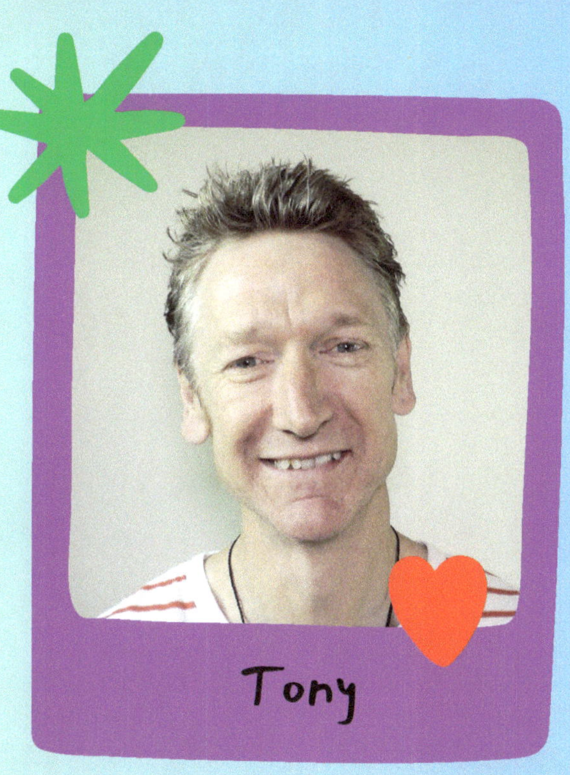

FUN ACTIVITIES!

Here are some fun activities that cross the midline.

These can be done at home, in the classroom, in a clinic, one-on-one, or in small groups.

RAINBOWS

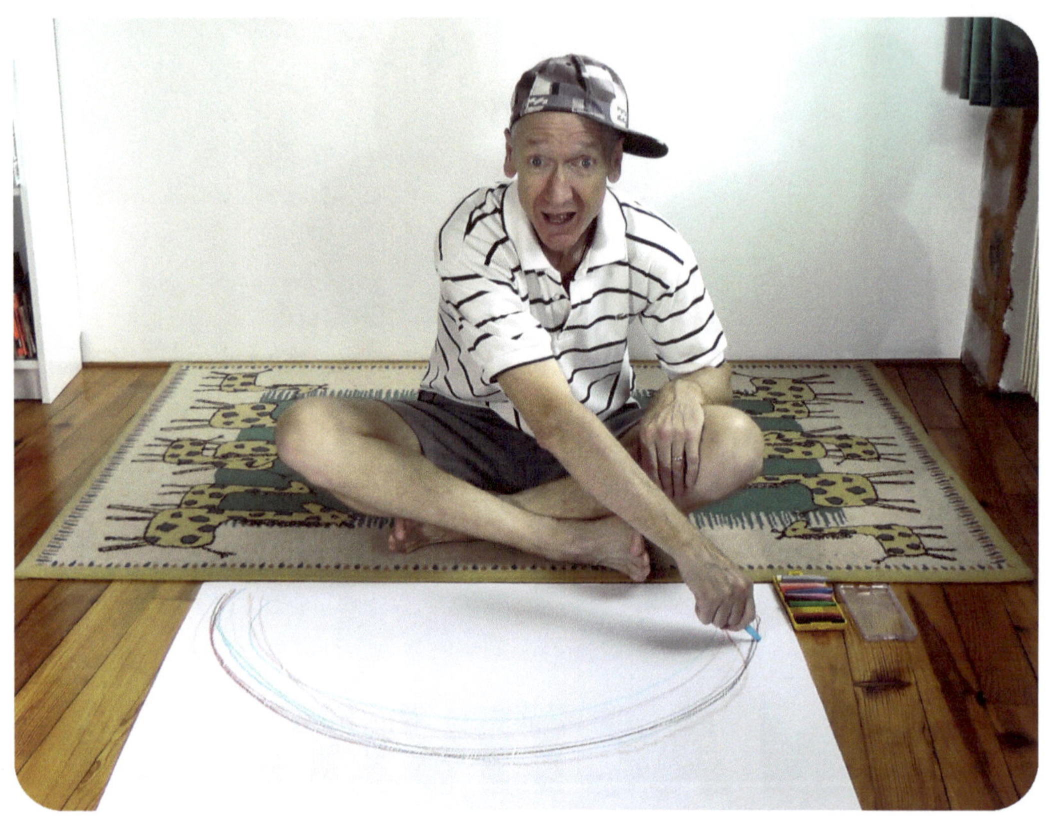

1. Stick a large piece of newsprint paper on the floor.
2. Your friend sits in front of or on the paper with coloured pencils, crayons etc.
3. Ask your friend to draw a rainbow. They must draw different coloured arches, starting from one side of the paper, crossing the midline, and over to the other side of the paper.
4. If needed, you can help by drawing start and finish points on each side.

TIDY UP, TONY!

Tony has made a terrible mess. Can you help him tidy up?

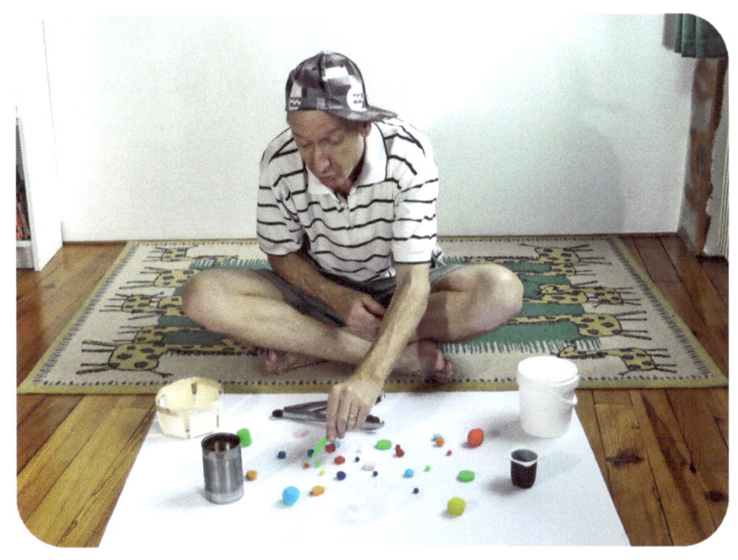

1. Place empty containers *(bowls, pots, cans, cups, etc.)* in the shape of an arch on the floor.
2. Place your friend in the middle of the arch.
3. Give your friend a pair of tongs or tweezers.
4. Now randomly scatter household objects all around your friend. Be sure to go to the sides and a little behind. *You can use cotton balls, beads, toys, Lego etc.*
5. Your friend must use the tongs/tweezers to pick up individual objects and place them into the containers. You choose what goes where.

TIME CHALLENGE VARIATION

You can time your friend! How long does it take to tidy up Tony's mess?
Or perhaps give your friend 60 seconds to tidy as much as possible.

This activity is an old, schoolground favourite that crosses the midline with arms and hands.

1. Sit down in front of your friend, on the floor or somewhere comfortable and recite the rhyme "Peas Porridge Hot".
2. While reciting the rhyme and in time with the rhyme, do the clapping motions. *These motions cross the midline.*

"Peas Porridge Hot"

Peas porridge hot.
Peas porridge cold.
Peas porridge in the pot,
Nine days old.

Some like it hot.
Some like it cold.
Some like it in the pot,
Nine days old!

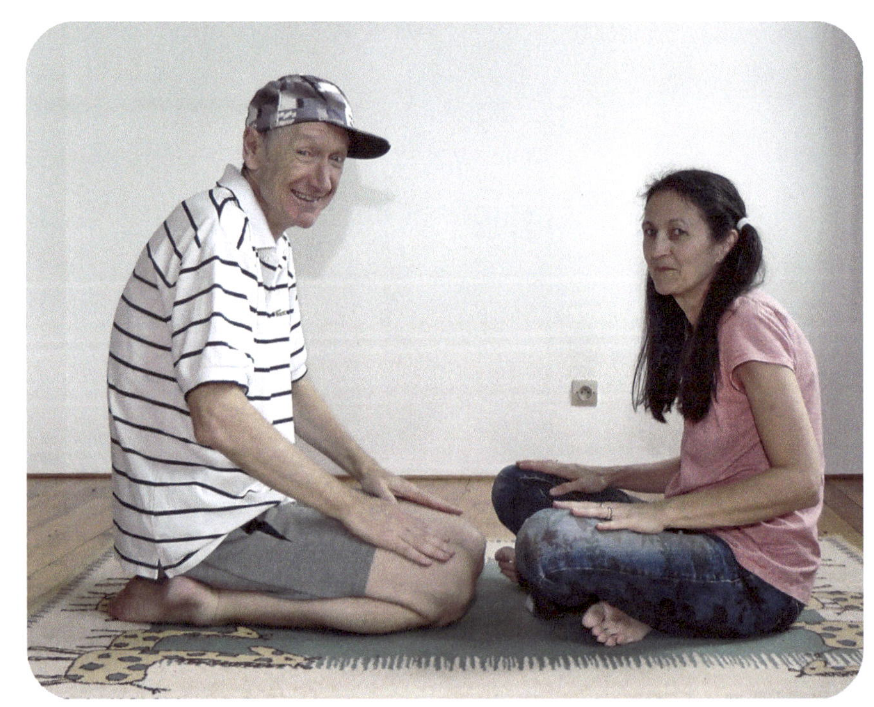

PEAS PORRIDGE HOT ACTIONS
VERSES 1 & 2

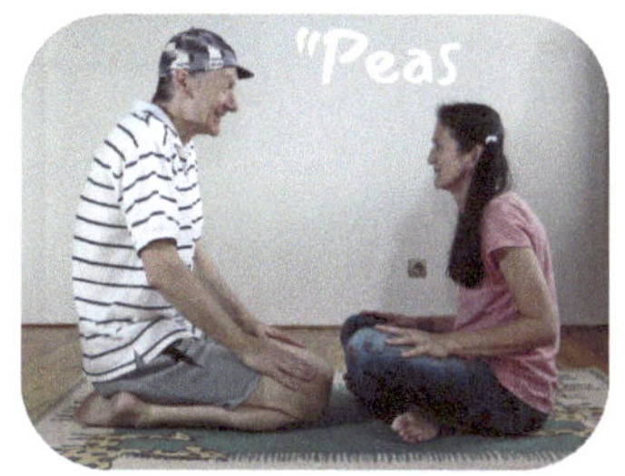

(clap both hands to thighs)

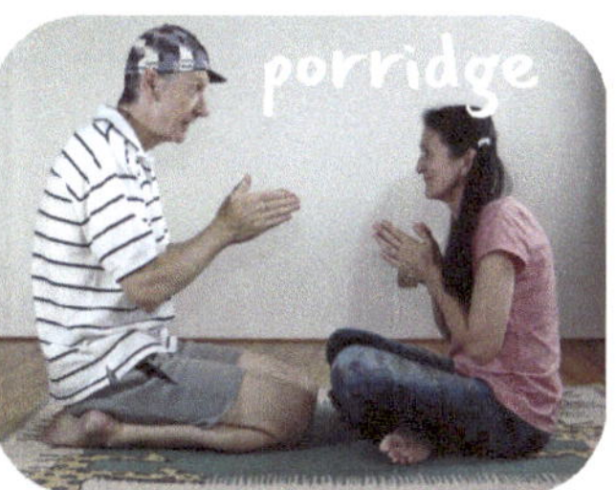

(clap own hands together)

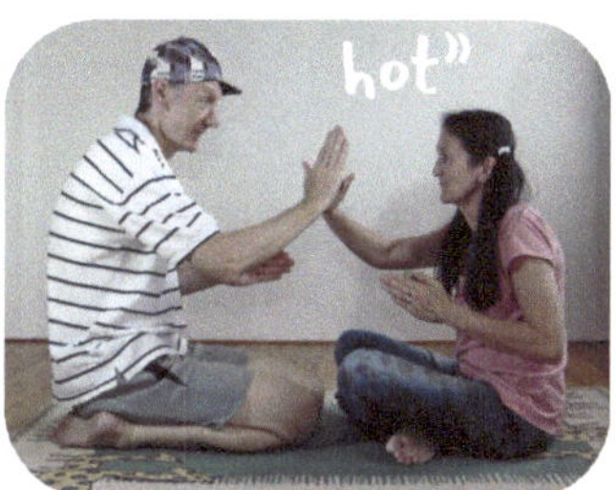

(clap partner's right hand)

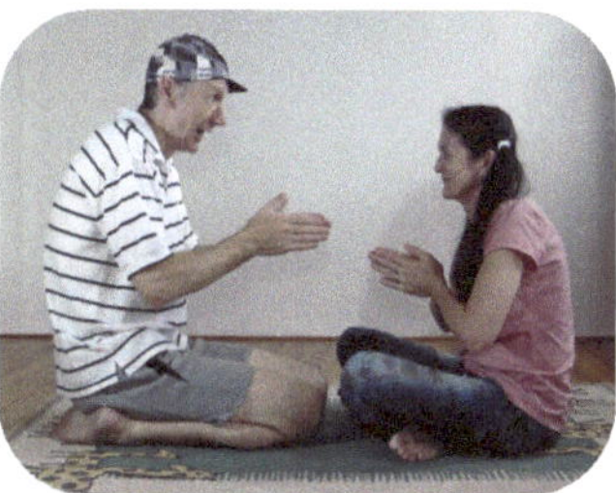
(clap own hands together)

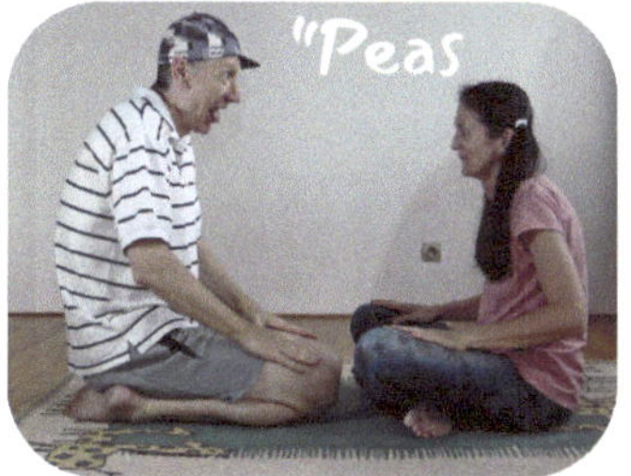

(clap both hands to thighs)

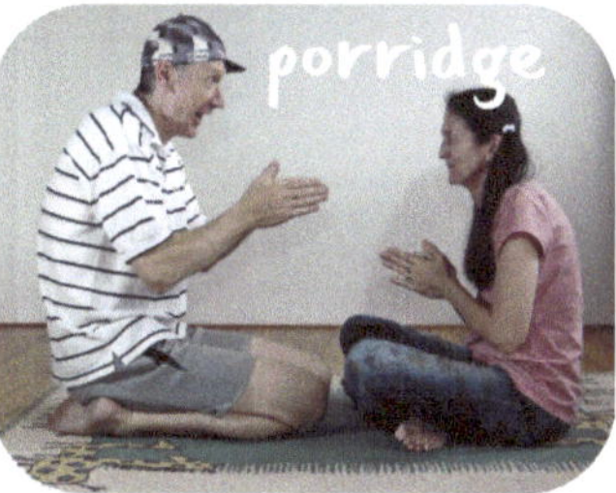

(clap own hands together)

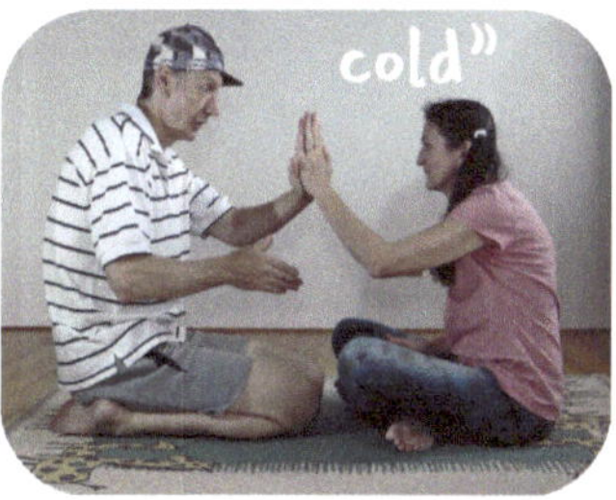

(clap partner's left hand)

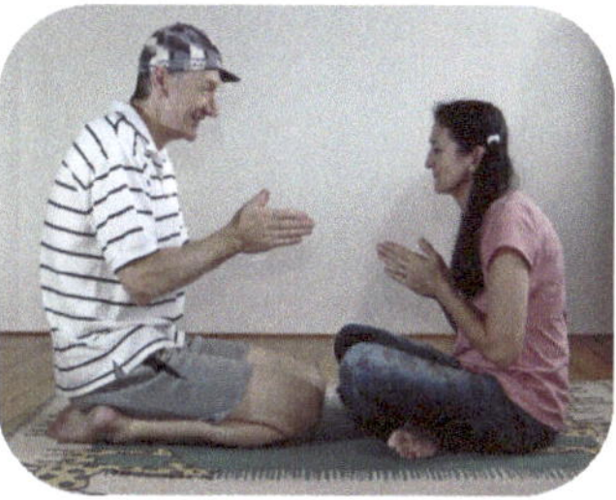
(clap own hands together),

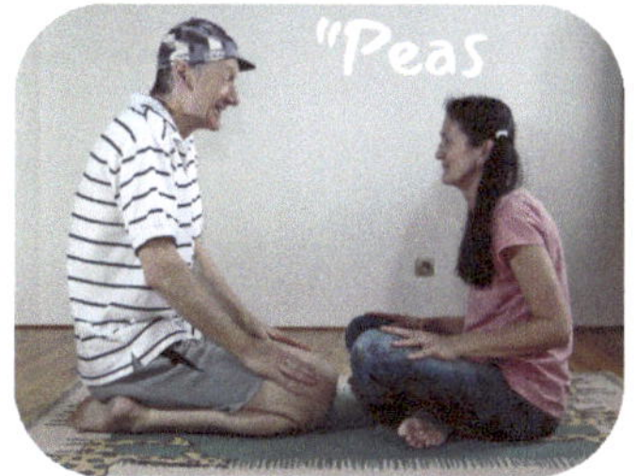

(clap both hands to thighs)

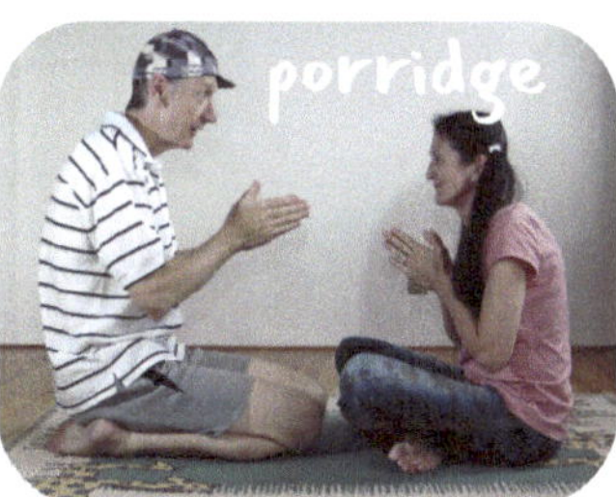

(clap own hands together)

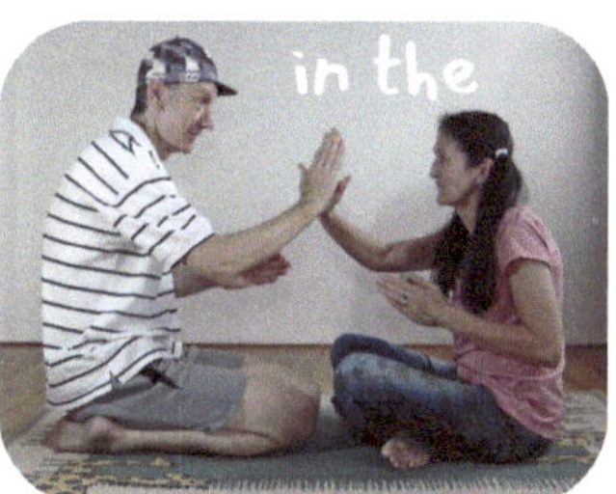

(clap partner's right hand)

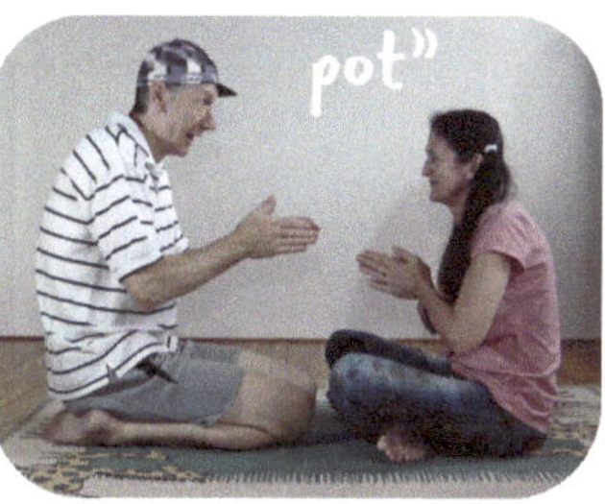

(clap own hands together),

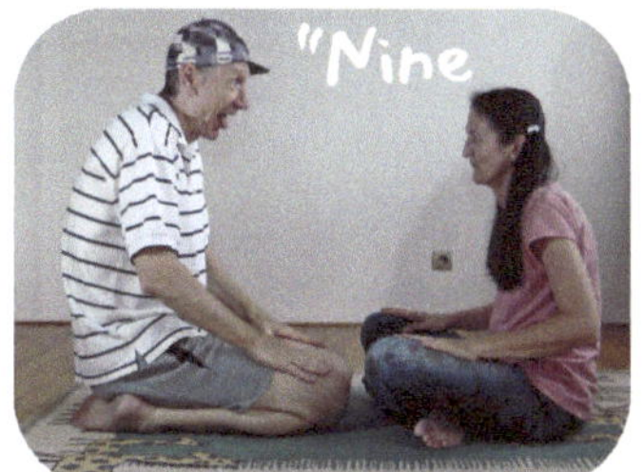

(clap both hands to thighs)

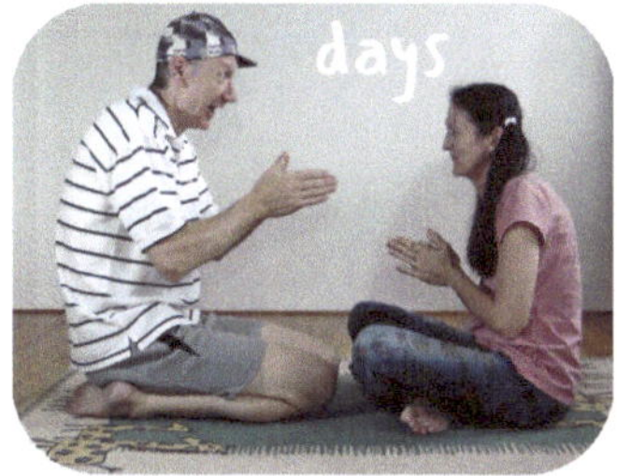

(clap own hands together)

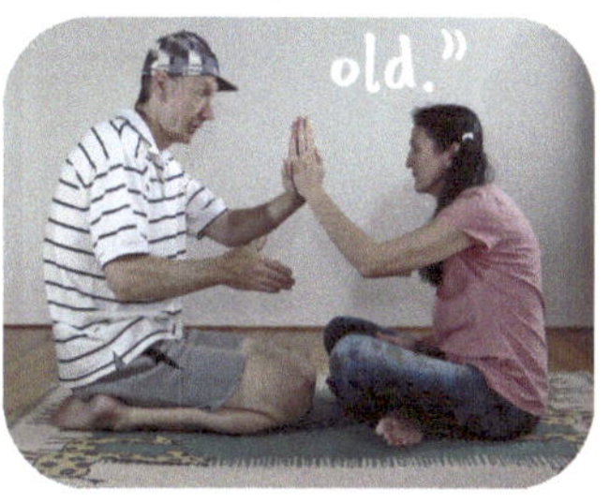

(clap partner's left hand)

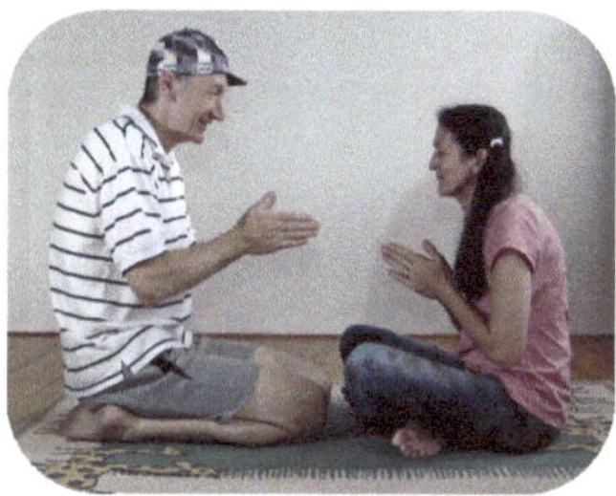
(clap own hands)

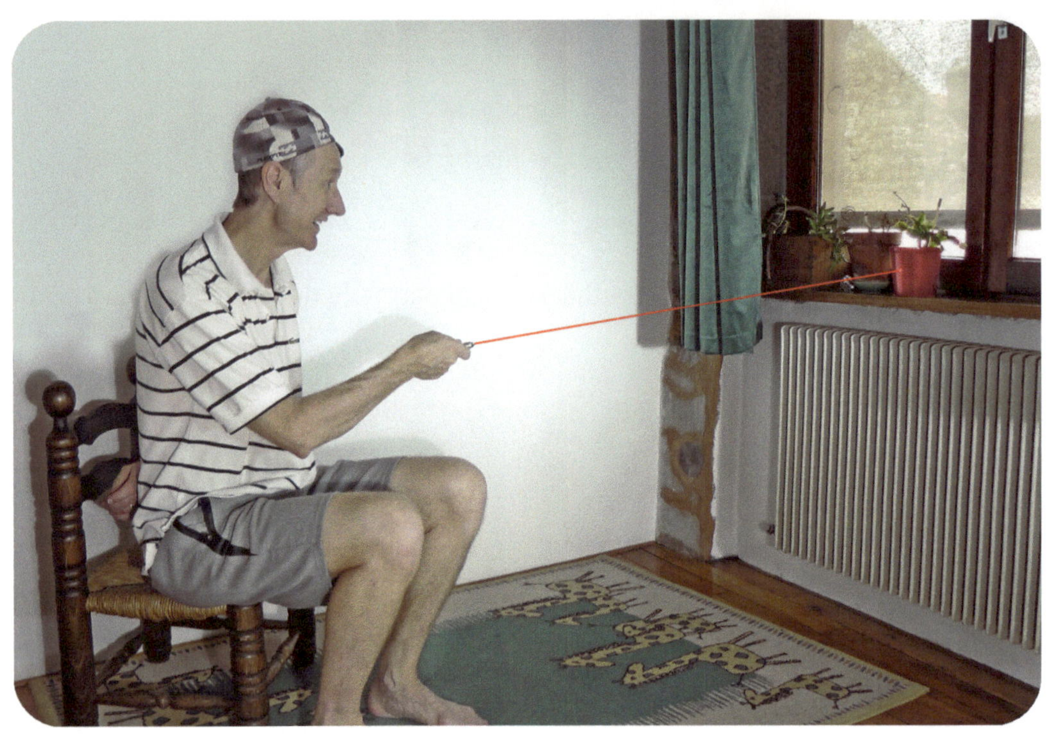

1. Ask your friend to sit in a chair.
2. Give your friend a laser pointer *(or a powerful torch)*.
3. Your friend must hold the laser pointer in one hand and **can only move this arm**.
4. Ask your friend to shine the laser pointer on objects around the room. *Be sure to make your friend cross the midline with their hand.*
5. Swap hands!

You can also play games like:
- *"I Spy With My Little Eye"*
- *"Find things that are blue"*

BALLOON TOUCH

1. Hold a balloon in front of your friend.
2. Ask your friend to touch the balloon with different body parts like the *first fingers, elbows, forehead, knees, feet, shoulders, and nose.*

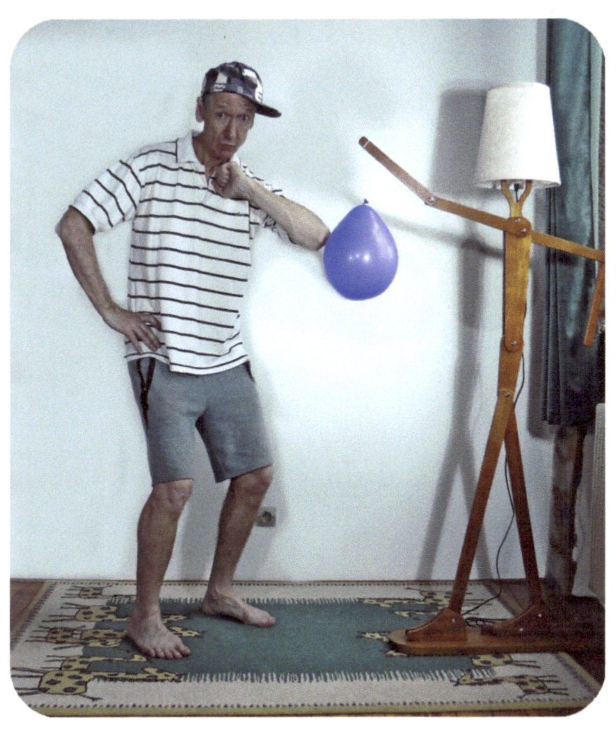 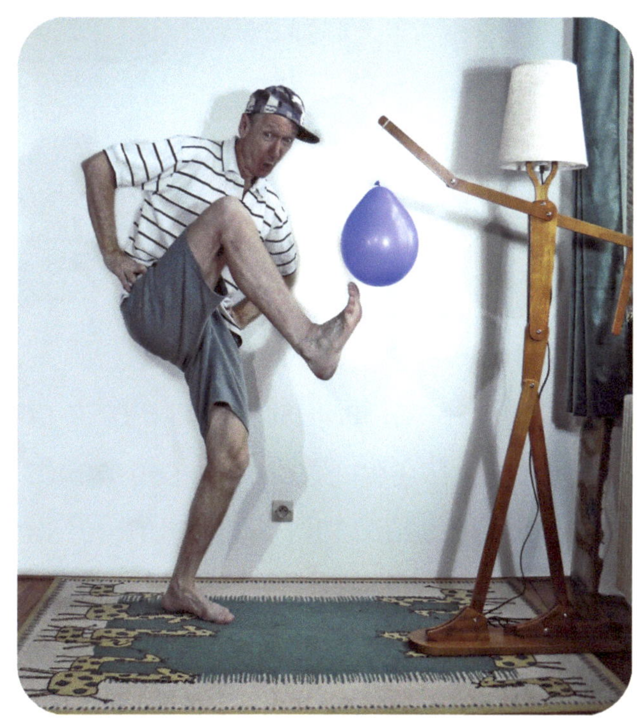

Now play **"Keep It Up"**.

1. Your friend must try to keep the balloon in the air by using only their first fingers and elbows or head, a knee and a foot.

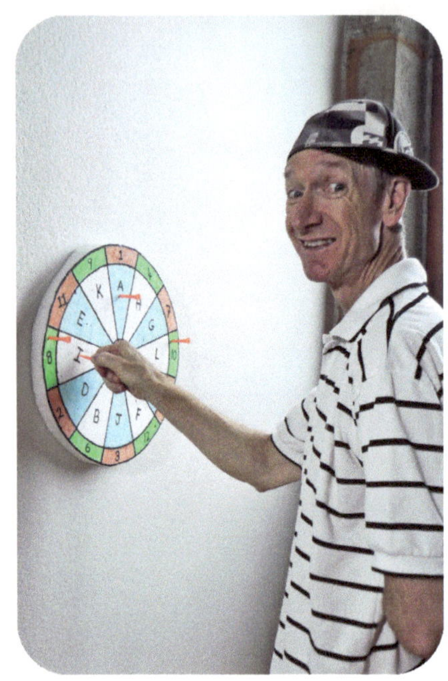

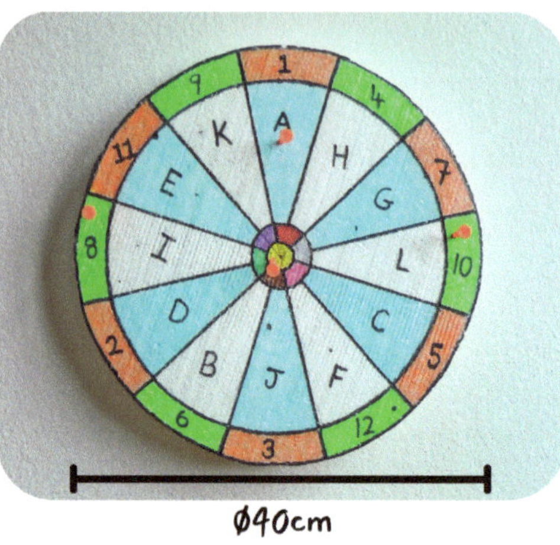

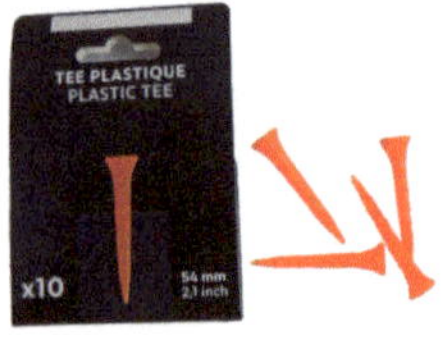

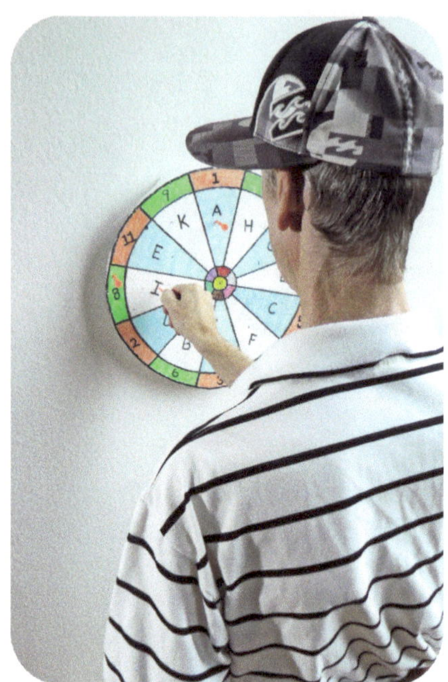

Build a polystyrene Dartboard

- *Cut a piece of polystyrene into a circle.*
- *Use felt tip pens to mark segments on the circle like a dart board.*
- *Label the segments with numbers and letters.*

1. Stick the dartboard to a wall.
2. Stand your friend in front of the dartboard, with a collection of golf tees.
3. Call out a number or letter on the dartboard.
4. Your friend must place a golf tee into that number/letter on the dartboard, **using only one hand**, left or right.
5. You can start in a clockwise direction, then go anti-clockwise, or call random numbers/letters. Don't forget to **swap hands!**

FUN EXERCISES!

Here are some fun exercises that Cross the Midline.
These can be done in the classroom, but are best to
do one-on-one, for safety reasons.
Some of them can be very challenging, so remember
to be supportive!

This is a great exercise for hand-eye coordination.

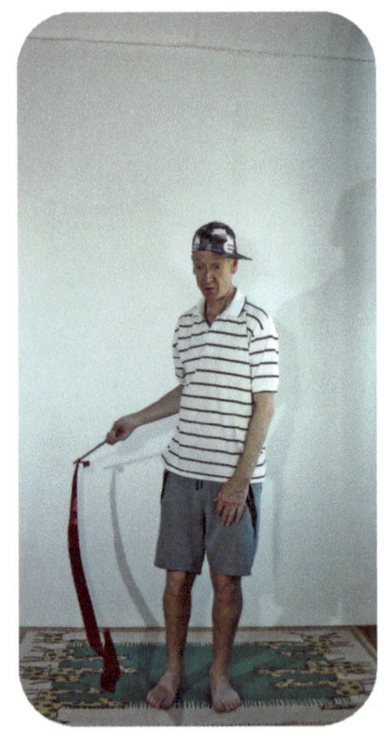 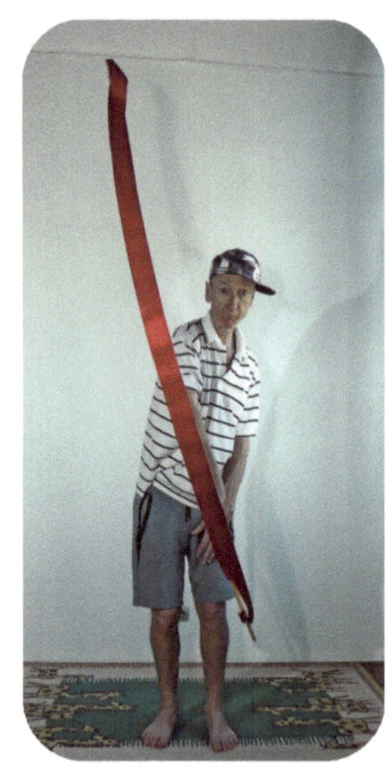 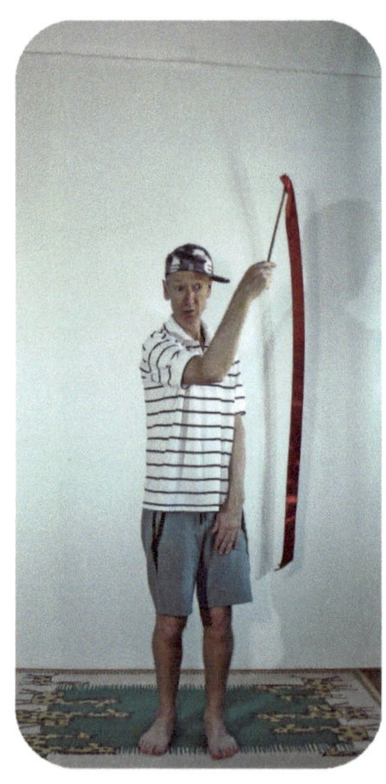

1. Attach a ribbon, streamer or several knotted scarves to the end of a length of dowel or a stick.
2. Holding the stick, ask your friend to swirl the ribbon overhead, from side to side, and up and down.
3. Give your friend a second ribbon stick, one in each hand.
4. Ask your friend to criss-cross the sticks in front of their face, alternating right and left arms.

Extra Challenge!

Use tape or rope to make a straight line on the floor.

Ask your friend to walk along the line, criss-crossing the ribbon sticks. Now backwards!

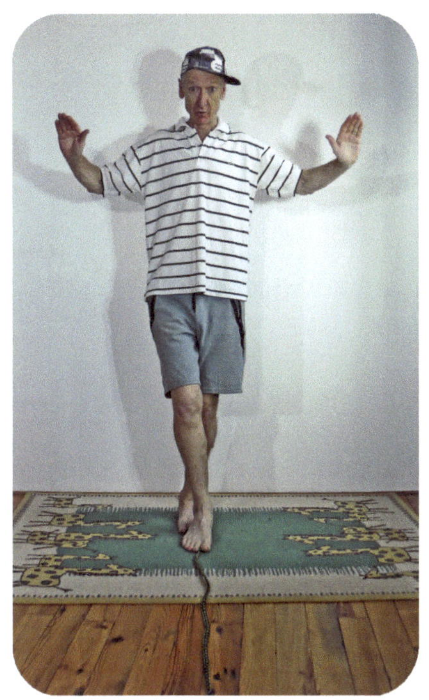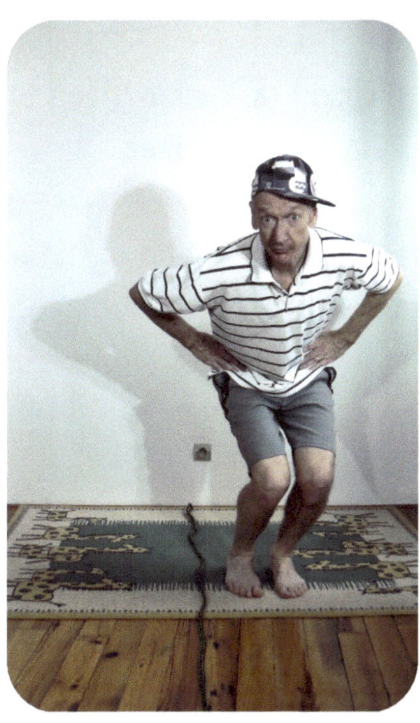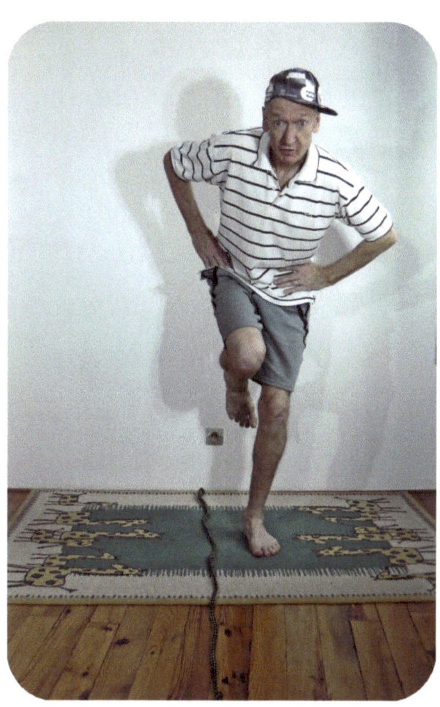

Create a 'balance beam' with a **length of rope**, 2–3 metres long.

Place the rope on the floor.

All exercises should be done **forward,** then **backward**.

To begin:

1. Ask your friend to **walk along** the rope, *one foot in front of the other.*
2. Ask your friend to **walk along** the rope, crossing from side to side, *one foot on one side, the other foot crosses over to the other side.*
3. Ask your friend to **jump across** the rope, *feet together.*
4. Ask your friend to **hop across** the rope.
5. Swap feet!

EXTRA CHALLENGE

To make exercises more and more difficult, ask your friend to **hold objects** in their hands *(like bean bags or ribbon sticks)* **as they do the exercises**.

1. Ask your friend to **toss** an object from one hand to the other as they do the exercise.
2. Place a **bucket** on one side of the rope. Ask your friend to **drop an object** into the bucket as they do the exercise.
3. Then, they must turn around and drop another object into the bucket. *This will **force them** to cross the midline!*
4. Ask your friend to **swing ribbon sticks** across their body as they do an exercise.

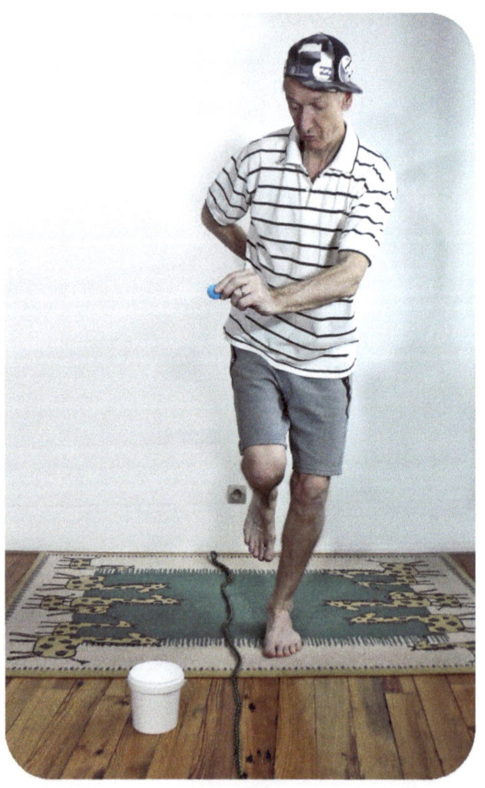

CRAWLING EXERCISES

These crawling exercises are physically difficult, so please be patient.
They develop the core muscles of the body along with left/right side coordination.
Because they are difficult, they take time.
Don't be overwhelmed by poor results when starting these exercises.
You will need a space at least 5m long.

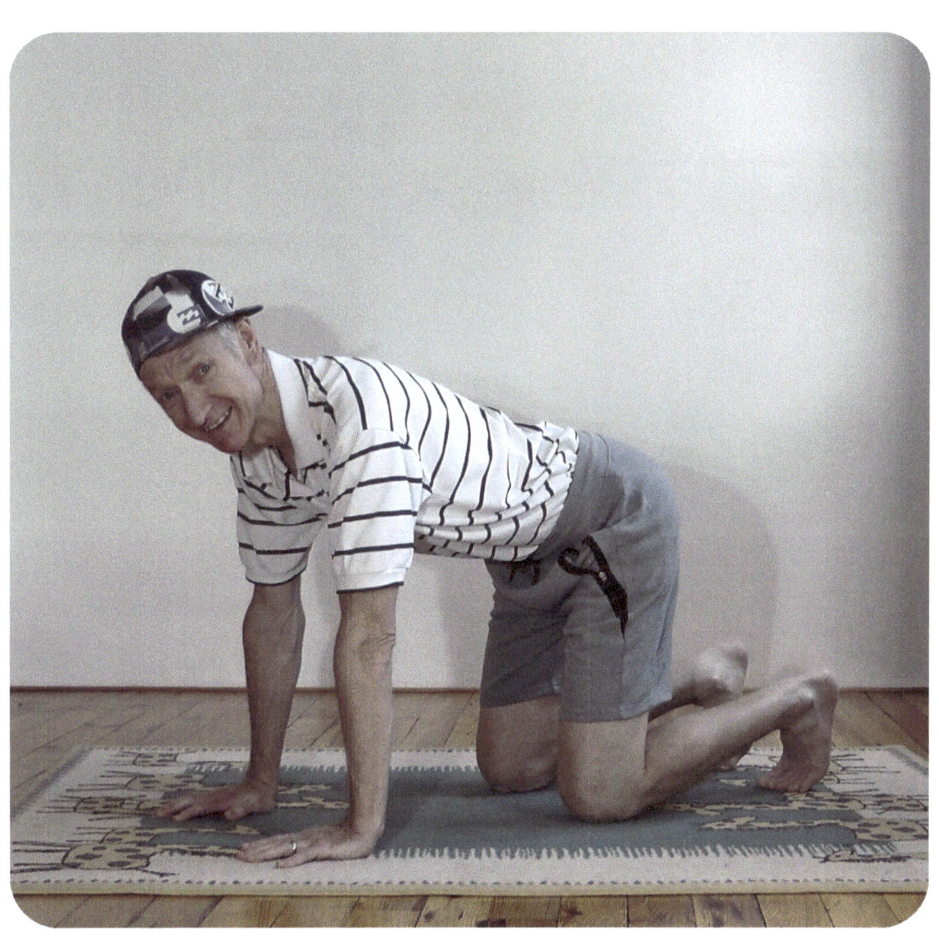

Bear Crawl

Remind your friend how we do the basic crawl: the **left arm** moves with the **right leg**, and the **right arm** moves with the **left leg.**

1. Start in the basic crawl position, back is straight, hands under shoulders and flat on the floor. Next, **lift your knees** up off the ground and begin to **crawl**.

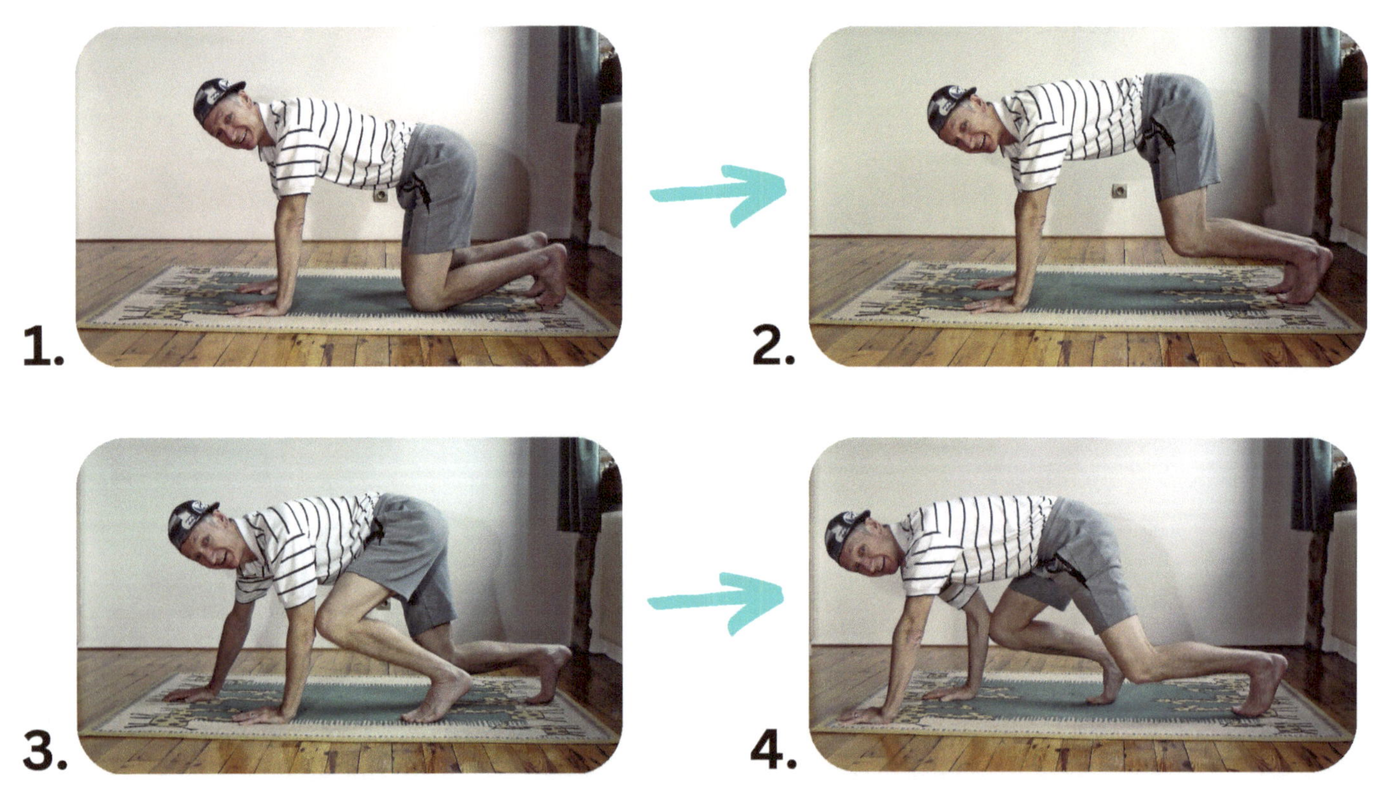

EXTRA CHALLENGE

Extend your hands just a little further forward and crawl.

Crocodile Crawl

The crocodile crawl is very hard, it's like a moving push-up! Don't worry if you can't go 5 metres, just go slowly and try to keep moving. It gets easier with time.

1. The starting position is just like for a push-up, with legs and arms shoulder-width apart.
2. Lower yourself down until your body is as low as you can be without touching the floor. **You need to keep as low as possible during the exercise.**
3. Begin crawling by bringing a knee forwards to an elbow, at the same time moving your opposite arm forward. Do the same for the other side.

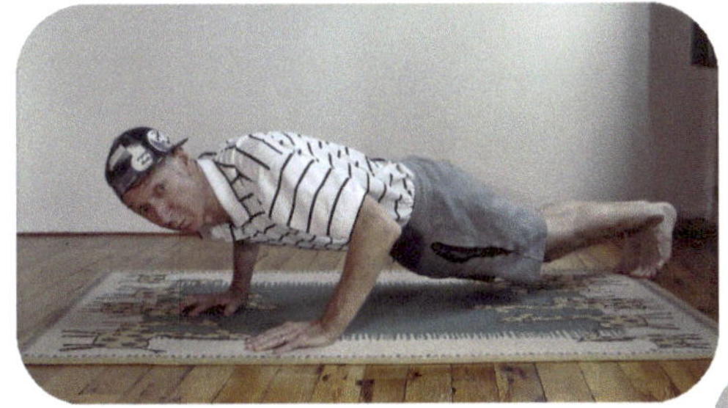
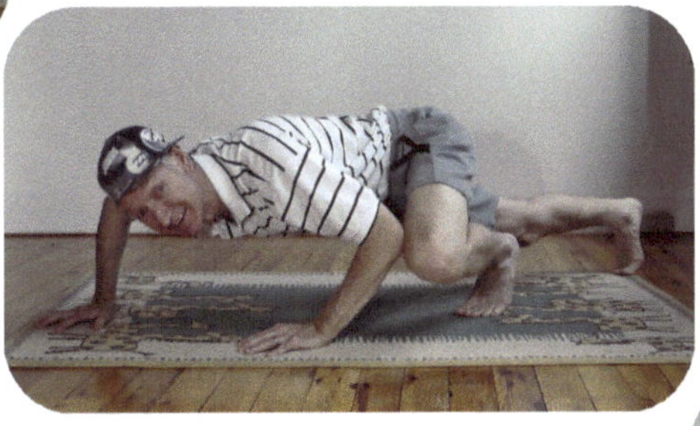
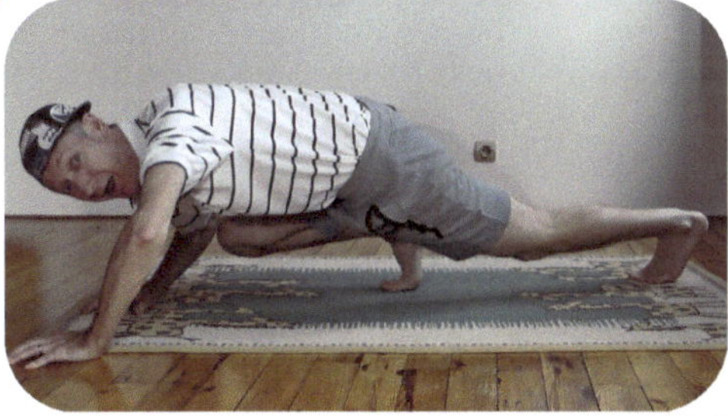

THANK YOU!

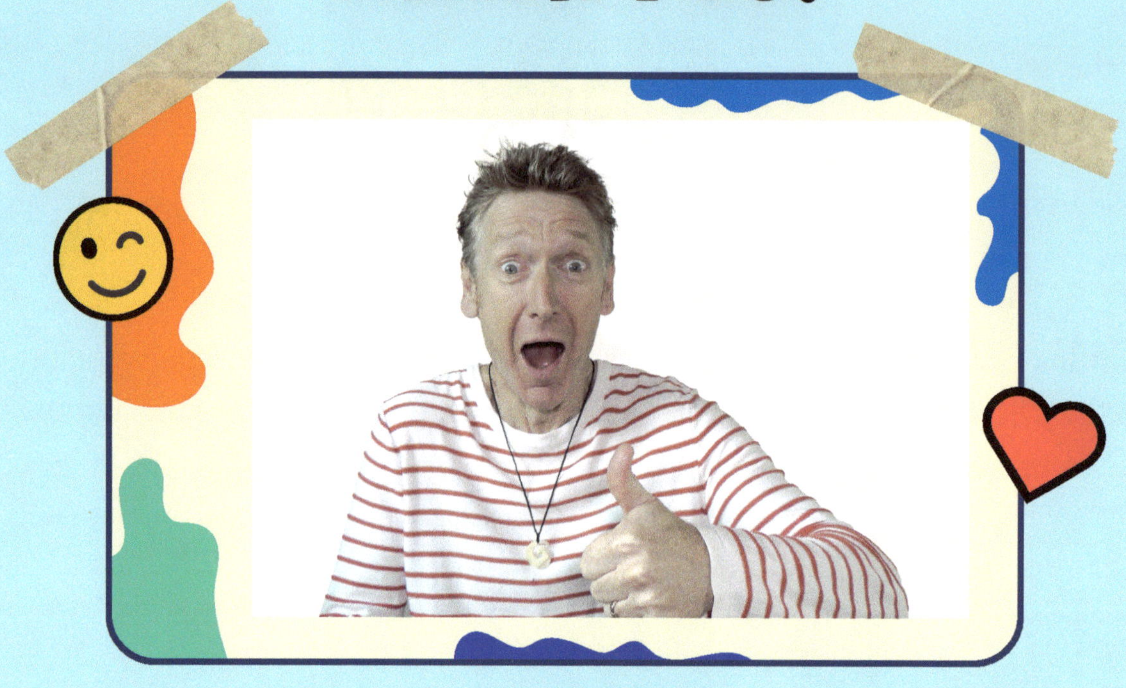

Hey, thanks for doing these dances, activities and exercises with me. I hope you had fun crossing the midline. Keep up the great work!

If you would like to get in touch you can sign-up for news on my website here: https://singalongwithtony.com/join-the-community/

If you're looking for educational songs and nursary rhymes you can check out my YouTube channel or follow me on Spotify !

Bye for now!
Tony

Credits

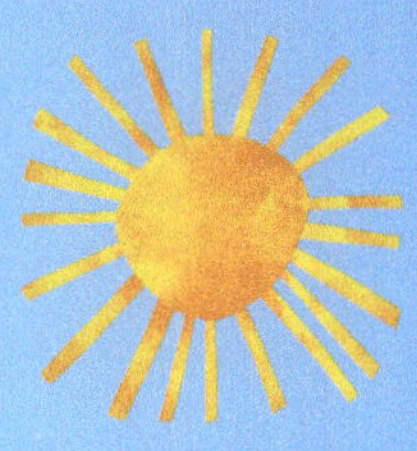

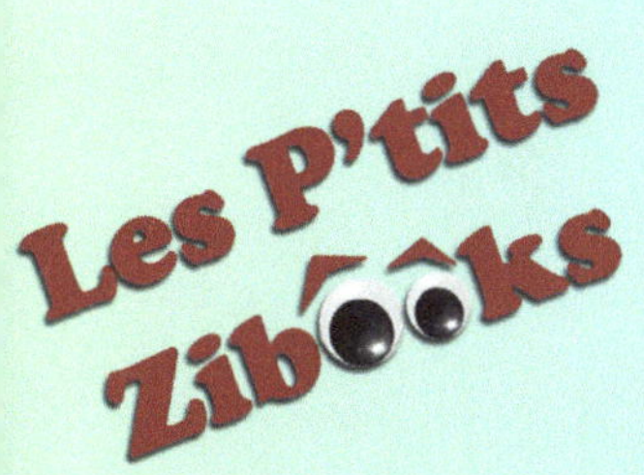

"Les Ptits Zibooks" by **Pascale Rival** are a magnificent collection of e-books that teach languages to primary school children throughout France. They offer a turnkey solution to help non-specialist teachers.

Sing Along With Tony's album "Little Carrot's Friends" was written especially for this wonderful product!

Tony Wyeth is the creative force behind **Sing Along With Tony**, a fun, musical way to learn. Beginning life as a musical theatre show that toured France, Sing Along With Tony offers live interactive performances and exciting new online resources for early childhood educators, primary schools and ESOL.

"Children's language and physical development benefits so much when they are engaged and having fun with songs and music". - Tony Wyeth